THE ULTIMATE
GLYCEMIC LOAD COUNTER

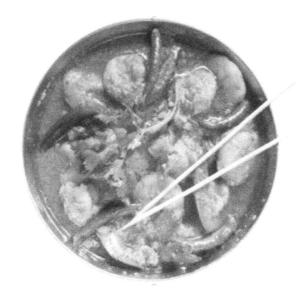

Discover Over 750 Low-Glycemic Foods, Along with Delicious Recipes for Healthy Eating.

DR. LINDA B. ALLEN

Copyright©2023 by Aria G James

All rights reserved. No part of this book may be reproduced, distributed, or transmitted in any form or by any means, including photocopying, recording, or other Electronic or mechanical methods, without the prior written permission of the author, except in the case of brief Quotations embodied in critical reviews and certain other Non-commercial uses permitted by copyright law. For Permission requests, write to the author, addressed "Attention: Permissions Coordinator."

DEDICATION

To the seekers of wellness and advocates of mindful nourishment, this comprehensive guide is dedicated.

It's dedicated to those who embark on a quest for better health through the choices they make at each meal. Your commitment to understanding the impact of food on your well-being inspires the pages within.

To my family and friends, your unwavering support and understanding throughout the creation of this guide have been invaluable. Your encouragement and belief in this mission have propelled its fruition.

Finally, to the readers, it's for you that these words have taken shape, a comprehensive dedication to fostering a holistic approach to nutrition, health, and the joy that comes from nourishing both body and spirit.

May this book stand as a beacon, offering guidance, knowledge, and empowerment as you navigate the seas of mindful eating, making informed choices, and embracing a lifestyle abundant with well-being.

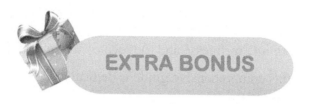

EXTRA BONUS

BONUS 1:

7-DAY

MEAL PLAN

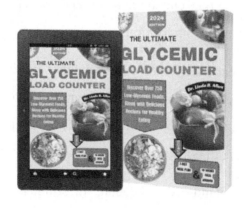

BONUS 2:

10-WEEKS

MEAL JOURNAL

TABLE OF CONTENTS

INTRODUCTION

In the hustle of modern life, our relationship with food often becomes a complex dance between convenience and health. We strive to nourish ourselves while navigating a maze of conflicting dietary advice. It was during one such journey through the labyrinth of nutrition that Victoria found herself at a crossroads.

Victoria, a spirited soul with a penchant for adventure, was navigating a maze of health challenges. Her quest for wellness led her to discover the pivotal concept of Glycemic Load. It was a eureka moment that transformed her approach to food.

Picture this: Victoria, a young professional juggling deadlines and responsibilities, found herself on a rollercoaster of energy crashes and mood swings. She longed for sustainable vitality, not fleeting bursts of energy from sugar-laden snacks. Enter Glycemic Load - a revelation that reshaped her understanding of how food impacts energy levels and overall health.

Intrigued and inspired, Victoria embarked on a quest to demystify Glycemic Load. Her journey led her through bustling markets, scientific journals, and conversations with experts. Along the way, she encountered a plethora of low-Glycemic foods that promised sustained energy and vitality.

"The Ultimate Glycemic Load Counter" is a culmination of Victoria's odyssey, an inclusive roadmap for anyone seeking a harmonious relationship between food and well-being.

Join us on this expedition, a journey beyond the confines of diets and restrictions, towards a lifestyle that celebrates both health and flavor. Let's embark together on a quest for sustained vitality, one nourishing meal at a time.

Welcome to a world where food is not just sustenance but a catalyst for a vibrant life.

Understanding Glycemic Load And Its Impact on Health

Unraveling the Glycemic Load Puzzle

In the intricate world of nutrition, understanding the nuances of Glycemic Load (GL) stands as a pivotal cornerstone in achieving optimal health and well-being. It goes beyond simply categorizing foods as "good" or "bad" but delves into the complex interplay between carbohydrates, blood sugar levels, and their subsequent impact on our bodies.

What is Glycemic Load?

Glycemic Load represents a refined measurement that evaluates how a specific portion of food affects blood sugar levels after consumption. Unlike the Glycemic Index (GI), which solely examines the impact of carbohydrates on blood sugar, Glycemic Load considers both the quality and quantity of carbohydrates in a given serving of food.

The Formula Behind Glycemic Load

The calculation of Glycemic Load involves multiplying a food's Glycemic Index by its carbohydrate content per serving and dividing that number by 100. This formula offers a more comprehensive view by considering not only how quickly a carbohydrate is metabolized but also the actual amount of carbohydrates presents in a typical portion.

Glycemic Load in Context: A Practical Understanding

Understanding Glycemic Load isn't just about numbers, it's about practical application. Foods with a high Glycemic Load tend to cause rapid spikes in blood sugar levels, followed by crashes, leading to fluctuations in energy and potential long-term health implications. Conversely, foods with a low Glycemic Load are digested and absorbed more slowly, providing a gradual release of energy and maintaining stable blood sugar levels.

Impact on Health and Well-Being

The implications of Glycemic Load on health are profound. High-Glycemic Load diets have been associated with an increased risk of type 2 diabetes, obesity, cardiovascular diseases, and even certain cancers. Understanding and managing Glycemic Load can aid in blood sugar management, weight control, and reducing the risk of chronic diseases, thereby promoting overall health and vitality.

How Glycemic Load Differs from Glycemic Index

Unpacking the Glycemic Index vs. Glycemic Load Debate

While Glycemic Load and Glycemic Index share a common ground in assessing the impact of carbohydrates on blood sugar levels, they represent distinct approaches in understanding this influence.

Glycemic Index: A Snapshot of Carbohydrate Impact

The Glycemic Index measures how quickly a particular carbohydrate-containing food raises blood sugar levels compared to pure glucose (which has a GI of 100). It serves as a relative ranking system, categorizing foods as high, moderate, or low in their ability to raise blood sugar levels.

Glycemic Index Limitations

However, the Glycemic Index has limitations, it doesn't account for the quantity of carbohydrates consumed. For instance, watermelon has a high GI, but the actual Glycemic Load per serving is relatively low due to its low carbohydrate content per serving. This distinction becomes crucial in practical dietary considerations.

Glycemic Load: The Comprehensive Picture

Glycemic Load fills the gaps left by the Glycemic Index by factoring in both the quality and quantity of carbohydrates in a given portion. This nuanced approach provides a more accurate representation of how a food affects blood sugar levels and offers practical guidance for meal planning and dietary choices.

Practical Application and Decision-Making

Understanding the difference between Glycemic Load and Glycemic Index is vital in making informed food choices. While the Glycemic Index provides a snapshot, the Glycemic Load offers a more comprehensive view, guiding individuals towards selecting foods that not only have a lower impact on blood sugar levels but also promote sustained energy and overall health.

In the ongoing quest for optimal health and well-being, comprehending the intricacies of Glycemic Load and its differentiation from Glycemic Index emerges as a crucial step. Armed with this knowledge, individuals can navigate the dietary landscape with clarity, making informed choices that contribute to sustained vitality and overall wellness.

BASICS OF GLYCEMIC LOAD

Unveiling the Core Concepts

In the realm of nutrition, the term "Glycemic Load" (GL) serves as a fundamental metric that goes beyond the simple classification of carbohydrates. Understanding the intricacies of Glycemic Load is key to making informed dietary choices for optimal health and well-being.

Explaining Glycemic Load in Detail

While Glycemic Index (GI) classifies carbohydrates based on their immediate impact on blood sugar levels, Glycemic Load offers a more comprehensive view. It not only considers the quality of carbohydrates but also the quantity present in a typical serving of food.

The Calculation: Unveiling the Formula

The formula for Glycemic Load involves multiplying a food's Glycemic Index by its carbohydrate content per serving, then dividing that number by 100. This method factors in both the rate of carbohydrate metabolism and the actual amount of carbohydrates consumed, providing a more accurate assessment of a food's impact on blood sugar levels.

Practical Implications of Glycemic Load

Foods with a high Glycemic Load tend to cause rapid spikes in blood sugar levels, leading to energy crashes and potential long-term health complications. Conversely, foods with a low Glycemic Load are digested more slowly, leading to a gradual release of energy and maintaining stable blood sugar levels.

Understanding the Dynamics of Carbohydrates

Carbohydrates serve as the primary source of energy for the body, but not all carbohydrates are created equal. The type and structure of carbohydrates influence how quickly they are broken down and absorbed in the bloodstream, ultimately impacting blood sugar levels.

Influence of Carbohydrate Type

Simple carbohydrates, such as those found in sugary treats or refined grains, are quickly digested and cause rapid spikes in blood sugar levels, contributing to a high Glycemic Load. On the other hand, complex carbohydrates, like those in whole grains, legumes, and fibrous vegetables, are digested more slowly, resulting in a lower Glycemic Load.

Role of Fiber and Fat

The presence of fiber and fat in a meal can also influence Glycemic Load. Fiber slows down the digestion and absorption of carbohydrates, reducing their impact on blood sugar levels. Similarly, the inclusion of healthy fats can further slowdown digestion, contributing to a lower Glycemic Load.

Factors Influencing Glycemic Load of Foods

Quantity of Carbohydrates

The total amount of carbohydrates in a serving of food significantly impacts its Glycemic Load. Even if a food has a relatively high Glycemic Index, consuming a smaller portion can result in a lower Glycemic Load.

Processing and Cooking Methods

The degree of processing and cooking methods can alter the Glycemic Load of foods. For instance, cooking pasta al dente reduces its Glycemic Load compared to overcooking it, as it slows down the digestion process.

Food Pairings and Combinations

Combining high-Glycemic Load foods with low-Glycemic Load foods can moderate the overall Glycemic Load of a meal. Pairing a high-Glycemic food with protein, fiber, or healthy fats can slow down digestion, mitigating the spike in blood sugar levels.

Importance of Glycemic Load in Diet Planning

Blood Sugar Management

Understanding and managing Glycemic Load play a crucial role in blood sugar management, particularly for individuals with diabetes or insulin resistance. Choosing foods with a lower Glycemic Load can help stabilize blood sugar levels and reduce the risk of complications.

Weight Management

Glycemic Load also influences weight management. Foods with a lower Glycemic Load tend to promote satiety and prevent overeating by providing sustained energy levels, aiding in weight control and potentially reducing the risk of obesity.

Long-Term Health Implications

Diets with a high Glycemic Load have been linked to an increased risk of chronic diseases such as type 2 diabetes, cardiovascular diseases, and metabolic syndrome. Incorporating low-Glycemic Load foods into the diet can contribute to long-term health and reduce the risk of these conditions.

Practical Applications in Diet Planning

Incorporating the principles of Glycemic Load into diet planning involves choosing a variety of nutrient-dense, low-Glycemic Load foods such as whole grains, legumes, fruits, and vegetables. Balancing meals with a mix of carbohydrates, proteins, healthy fats, and fiber can help manage Glycemic Load and promote overall health.

The understanding of Glycemic Load goes beyond mere categorization of foods, it provides a nuanced view of how different carbohydrates impact blood sugar levels. Armed with this knowledge, individuals can make informed dietary choices, optimizing their health, managing blood sugar levels, and promoting overall well-being.

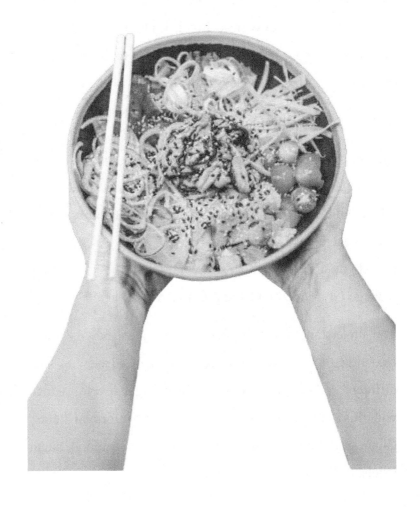

COMPREHENSIVE LIST OF LOW-GLYCEMIC FOODS

Non-Starchy Vegetables

Bell Peppers

GI: 10, GL: 1 (per 80g portion)

Preparation: Sliced, raw in salads or roasted with olive oil.

Broccoli

GI: 15, GL: 1 (per 80g portion)

Preparation: Steamed or lightly sautéed with garlic.

Cauliflower

GI: 10, GL: 1 (per 80g portion)

Preparation: Roasted with herbs and spices or mashed as a low-carb alternative to mashed potatoes.

Spinach

GI: 15, GL: 1 (per 80g portion)

Preparation: Raw in salads or lightly cooked in olive oil with garlic.

Zucchini

GI: 15, GL: 2 (per 80g portion)

Preparation: Spiralized as noodles or sautéed with herbs and a splash of lemon juice.

Asparagus

GI: 15, GL: 1 (per 80g portion)

Preparation: Grilled or roasted with a drizzle of olive oil and balsamic vinegar.

Cabbage

GI: 10, GL: 1 (per 80g portion)

Preparation: Shredded in coleslaw or stir-fried with other vegetables.

Brussels Sprouts

GI: 15, GL: 2 (per 80g portion)

Preparation: Roasted with a touch of olive oil and balsamic glaze.

Kale

GI: 15, GL: 1 (per 80g portion)

Preparation: Massaged with olive oil and used in salads or baked into kale chips.

Artichokes

GI: 15, GL: 1 (per medium-sized artichoke)

Preparation: Steamed and served with a light vinaigrette or roasted with garlic.

Cucumber

GI: 15, GL: 1 (per 80g portion)

Preparation: Sliced for salads or eaten raw as a snack with hummus.

Celery

GI: 15, GL: 1 (per 80g portion)

Preparation: Sliced and added to soups or used as a crunchy snack with nut butter.

Eggplant

GI: 15, GL: 2 (per 80g portion)

Preparation: Grilled or roasted and used in dishes like ratatouille or baba ganoush.

Mushrooms

GI: 10, GL: 1 (per 80g portion)

Preparation: Sautéed with garlic and herbs, or grilled as a side dish.

Green Beans

GI: 15, GL: 2 (per 80g portion)

Preparation: Steamed or blanched and served as a side dish or in salads.

Onions

GI: 10, GL: 1 (per 80g portion)

Preparation: Sautéed or caramelized to enhance flavor in various dishes.

Leeks

GI: 15, GL: 1 (per 80g portion)

Preparation: Sliced and added to soups or sautéed as a side dish.

Radishes

GI: 15, GL: 1 (per 80g portion)

Preparation: Sliced for salads or pickled as a crunchy addition to meals.

Snow Peas

GI: 15, GL: 2 (per 80g portion)

Preparation: Lightly stir-fried or added to stir-fries for crunch.

Turnips

GI: 15, GL: 1 (per 80g portion)

Preparation: Roasted or mashed as a lower-carb alternative to potatoes.

Fennel

GI: 15, GL: 1 (per 80g portion)

Preparation: Sliced thinly for salads or roasted with other vegetables.

Bok Choy

GI: 15, GL: 1 (per 80g portion)

Preparation: Stir-fried or steamed as a side dish.

Beets

GI: 15, GL: 2 (per 80g portion)

Preparation: Roasted or grated raw in salads.

Peppers (Hot)

GI: 15, GL: 1 (per 80g portion)

Preparation: Diced and added to dishes for heat or pickled for a spicy condiment.

Collard Greens

GI: 10, GL: 1 (per 80g portion)

Preparation: Sautéed or steamed as a side dish or added to soups.

Radicchio

GI: 15, GL: 1 (per 80g portion)

Preparation: Raw in salads or grilled for added flavor.

Chard

GI: 15

GL: 1 (per 80g portion)

Preparation: Sautéed with garlic and olive oil or added to soups.

Squash (Butternut)

GI: 15

GL: 2 (per 80g portion)

Preparation: Roasted and served as a side dish or pureed into soups.

Pumpkin

GI: 15, GL: 1 (per 80g portion)

Preparation: Roasted and used in soups, stews, or baked goods.

Okra

GI: 20, GL: 2 (per 80g portion)

Preparation: Lightly sautéed or roasted for a crispy texture.

Leafy Greens

Spinach

GI: 15, GL: 1 (per 80g portion)

Preparation: Raw in salads or lightly cooked in olive oil with garlic.

Kale

GI: 15, GL: 1 (per 80g portion)

Preparation: Massaged with olive oil and used in salads or baked into kale chips.

Arugula

GI: 15, GL: 1 (per 80g portion)

Preparation: Raw in salads with a drizzle of balsamic vinaigrette.

Swiss Chard

GI: 15

GL: 1 (per 80g portion)

Preparation: Sautéed with garlic and olive oil or added to soups.

Romaine Lettuce

GI: 15

GL: 1 (per 80g portion)

Preparation: Used as a base for salads or in lettuce wraps.

Collard Greens

GI: 10

GL: 1 (per 80g portion)

Preparation: Sautéed or steamed as a side dish or added to soups.

Turnip Greens

GI: 15

GL: 1 (per 80g portion)

Preparation: Sautéed with garlic or added to soups.

Mustard Greens

GI: 15

GL: 1 (per 80g portion)

Preparation: Sautéed or used in salads for a peppery flavor.

Beet Greens

GI: 15

GL: 1 (per 80g portion)

Preparation: Sautéed with garlic or added to soups for added nutrients.

Bok Choy

GI: 15

GL: 1 (per 80g portion)

Preparation: Stir-fried or steamed as a side dish.

Watercress

GI: 15

GL: 1 (per 80g portion)

Preparation: Raw in salads or used as a garnish for dishes.

Dandelion Greens

GI: 15

GL: 1 (per 80g portion)

Preparation: Raw in salads or lightly cooked with other greens.

Microgreens

GI: 15

GL: 1 (per 80g portion)

Preparation: Added to salads, sandwiches, or used as a garnish.

Endive

GI: 15

GL: 1 (per 80g portion)

Preparation: Raw in salads or used as a vessel for appetizers.

Sorrel

GI: 15

GL: 1 (per 80g portion)

Preparation: Raw in salads or used in soups for a tangy flavor.

Cabbage (Green)

GI: 10

GL: 1 (per 80g portion)

Preparation: Shredded in coleslaw or stir-fried with other vegetables.

Cabbage (Red)

GI: 10

GL: 1 (per 80g portion)

Preparation: Sliced for salads or lightly sautéed with other vegetables.

Iceberg Lettuce

GI: 15

GL: 1 (per 80g portion)

Preparation: Used in salads or as a wrap for fillings.

Radicchio

GI: 15

GL: 1 (per 80g portion)

Preparation: Raw in salads or grilled for added flavor.

Butter Lettuce

GI: 15

GL: 1 (per 80g portion)

Preparation: Used as a base for salads or in wraps.

Mizuna

GI: 15

GL: 1 (per 80g portion)

Preparation: Raw in salads or lightly sautéed.

Komatsuna

GI: 15

GL: 1 (per 80g portion)

Preparation: Stir-fried or added to soups for a mild flavor.

Amaranth Leaves

GI: 15

GL: 1 (per 80g portion)

Preparation: Cooked and used in various dishes like stews or sautés.

Chicory

GI: 15

GL: 1 (per 80g portion)

Preparation: Raw in salads or roasted as a side dish.

Kohlrabi Greens

GI: 15

GL: 1 (per 80g portion)

Preparation: Sautéed or added to soups for their mild flavor.

Chicory Greens

GI: 15

GL: 1 (per 80g portion)

Preparation: Used in salads or cooked as a side dish.

Rapini (Broccoli Rabe)

GI: 15

GL: 1 (per 80g portion)

Preparation: Sautéed with garlic and olive oil or added to pasta dishes.

Turnip Greens

GI: 15

GL: 1 (per 80g portion)

Preparation: Sautéed with garlic or added to soups.

African Kale (Sukuma Wiki)

GI: 15

GL: 1 (per 80g portion)

Preparation: Sautéed with onions and tomatoes or added to stews.

Lamb's Lettuce (Mâche)

GI: 15

GL: 1 (per 80g portion)

Cruciferous Vegetables

Cauliflower

GI: 10

GL: 1 (per 80g portion)

Preparation: Roasted with spices or mashed as a low-carb alternative.

Broccolini

GI: 15

GL: 1 (per 80g portion)

Preparation: Steamed and served as a side dish or added to stir-fries.

Kohlrabi

GI: 15

GL: 1 (per 80g portion)

Preparation: Sliced and eaten raw in salads or roasted with other vegetables.

Brussels Sprouts

GI: 15

GL: 2 (per 80g portion)

Preparation: Roasted with a touch of olive oil and balsamic glaze.

Bok Choy

GI: 15

GL: 1 (per 80g portion)

Preparation: Stir-fried or steamed as a side dish.

Radishes

GI: 15

GL: 1 (per 80g portion)

Preparation: Sliced for salads or pickled as a crunchy addition to meals.

Turnips

GI: 15

GL: 1 (per 80g portion)

Preparation: Roasted or mashed as a lower-carb alternative to potatoes.

Horseradish

GI: 15

GL: 1 (per 80g portion)

Preparation: Grated and used as a condiment or flavor enhancer in dishes.

Collard Greens

GI: 10

GL: 1 (per 80g portion)

Preparation: Sautéed or steamed as a side dish or added to soups.

Rutabaga

GI: 15

GL: 1 (per 80g portion)

Preparation: Roasted, mashed, or used in stews and soups.

Broccoli Rabe (Rapini)

GI: 15

GL: 1 (per 80g portion)

Preparation: Sautéed with garlic and olive oil or added to pasta dishes.

Garden Cress

GI: 15

GL: 1 (per 80g portion)

Preparation: Raw in salads or used as a garnish for dishes.

Chinese Broccoli (Gai Lan)

GI: 15

GL: 1 (per 80g portion)

Preparation: Steamed and served with a light soy sauce dressing.

Broccoflower

GI: 15

GL: 1 (per 80g portion)

Preparation: Roasted or steamed as a side dish.

Cabbage (Savoy)

GI: 10

GL: 1 (per 80g portion)

Preparation: Shredded in salads or stir-fried with other vegetables.

Chinese Cabbage (Napa)

GI: 15

GL: 1 (per 80g portion)

Preparation: Used in stir-fries or fermented for kimchi.

Broccoli Romanesco

GI: 15

GL: 1 (per 80g portion)

Preparation: Steamed or roasted with olive oil and herbs.

Leaf Mustard

GI: 15

GL: 1 (per 80g portion)

Preparation: Raw in salads or lightly cooked with other greens.

Kale Sprouts

GI: 15

GL: 1 (per 80g portion)

Preparation: Roasted or sautéed as a side dish.

Cauliflower Romanesco

GI: 10

GL: 1 (per 80g portion)

Preparation: Roasted with spices or used in salads.

Bok Choy (Baby)

GI: 15

GL: 1 (per 80g portion)

Preparation: Steamed or added to soups and stir-fries.

Daikon Radish

GI: 15

GL: 1 (per 80g portion)

Preparation: Sliced for salads or pickled as a side dish.

Chinese Mustard Greens

GI: 15

GL: 1 (per 80g portion)

Preparation: Sautéed or added to stir-fries for a peppery flavor.

Choy Sum

GI: 15

GL: 1 (per 80g portion)

Preparation: Steamed or stir-fried as a side dish.

Pak Choi

GI: 15

GL: 1 (per 80g portion)

Preparation: Stir-fried or added to soups for a mild flavor.

Gai Choy (Chinese Mustard Cabbage)

GI: 15

GL: 1 (per 80g portion)

Preparation: Sautéed or used in stir-fries and soups.

Black Kale (Cavolo Nero)

GI: 15

GL: 1 (per 80g portion)

Preparation: Massaged in salads or lightly cooked as a side dish.

Siberian Kale

GI: 15

GL: 1 (per 80g portion)

Preparation: Used in salads or lightly cooked with other greens.

White Cabbage

GI: 10

GL: 1 (per 80g portion)

Preparation: Shredded for coleslaw or cooked in various dishes.

Purple Kohlrabi

GI: 15

GL: 1 (per 80g portion)

Preparation: Sliced and eaten raw in salads or added to stir-fries.

Root Vegetables

Sweet Potato

GI: 70

GL: 17 (per 150g portion)

Preparation: Baked or roasted as fries, mashed, or added to soups and stews.

Carrot

GI: 47

GL: 3 (per 80g portion)

Preparation: Raw as a snack, grated in salads, or roasted with herbs.

Beetroot

GI: 61

GL: 5 (per 80g portion)

Preparation: Roasted, grated raw in salads, or used to make beetroot soup.

Parsnip

GI: 97

GL: 12 (per 80g portion)

Preparation: Roasted as a side dish or pureed in soups.

Rutabaga

GI: 72

GL: 4 (per 80g portion)

Preparation: Roasted, mashed, or used in stews and soups.

Turnip

GI: 55

GL: 3 (per 80g portion)

Preparation: Roasted, mashed, or added to soups and stews.

Yam

GI: 54

GL: 23 (per 150g portion)

Preparation: Baked, boiled, or used in casseroles and curries.

Celeriac

GI: 50

GL: 5 (per 80g portion)

Preparation: Mashed, roasted, or used in soups and stews.

Jicama

GI: 52

GL: 3 (per 80g portion)

Preparation: Sliced and eaten raw in salads or with dips.

Jerusalem Artichoke

GI: 50

GL: 3 (per 80g portion)

Preparation: Roasted, sautéed, or used in soups and stews.

Kohlrabi

GI: 50

GL: 2 (per 80g portion)

Preparation: Sliced and eaten raw in salads or roasted as a side dish.

Parsley Root

GI: 50

GL: 2 (per 80g portion)

Preparation: Roasted, added to soups or stews, or mashed.

Skirret

GI: 50

GL: 2 (per 80g portion)

Preparation: Cooked and used in various dishes like stews or soups.

Lotus Root

GI: 45

GL: 5 (per 80g portion)

Preparation: Sliced and stir-fried, used in soups, or pickled.

Cassava

GI: 46

GL: 10 (per 80g portion)

Preparation: Boiled, fried as chips, or used in stews and curries.

Water Chestnut

GI: 60

GL: 4 (per 80g portion)

Preparation: Sliced and used in stir-fries or salads.

Ginger

GI: 15

GL: 0 (per 80g portion)

Preparation: Used as a spice in various dishes or brewed as tea.

Turmeric

GI: 15

GL: 0 (per 80g portion)

Preparation: Used as a spice in curries, soups, and golden milk.

Arrowroot

GI: 65

GL: 12 (per 80g portion)

Preparation: Used as a thickening agent in sauces and soups.

Fennel Bulb

GI: 30

GL: 1 (per 80g portion)

Preparation: Sliced raw in salads or roasted with other vegetables.

Radish (Daikon)

GI: 15

GL: 1 (per 80g portion)

Preparation: Sliced for salads or pickled as a side dish.

Taro

GI: 55

GL: 8 (per 80g portion)

Preparation: Boiled, mashed, or used in curries and stews.

Scorzonera

GI: 35

GL: 1 (per 80g portion)

Preparation: Cooked and used in various dishes like stews or gratins.

Yautia (Malanga)

GI: 55

GL: 10 (per 80g portion)

Preparation: Boiled, mashed, or used in soups and stews.

Ramps (Wild Leeks)

GI: 35

GL: 1 (per 80g portion)

Preparation: Used in salads, pesto, or sautéed as a side dish.

Salsify

GI: 50

GL: 2 (per 80g portion)

Preparation: Cooked and used in various dishes like stews or soups.

Sweet Turnip

GI: 75

GL: 10 (per 80g portion)

Preparation: Roasted, mashed, or used in stews and soups.

Chinese Water Chestnut

GI: 60

GL: 3 (per 80g portion)

Preparation: Sliced and used in stir-fries or salads.

Yacon

GI: 40

GL: 1 (per 80g portion)

Preparation: Eaten raw, sliced in salads or used in smoothies.

Sunchoke

GI: 50

GL: 3 (per 80g portion)

Preparation: Roasted, sautéed, or used in soups and stews.

Berries

Strawberries

GI: 40

GL: 1 (per 80g portion)

Preparation: Eaten fresh, added to salads, or used in smoothies.

Blueberries

GI: 53

GL: 5 (per 80g portion)

Preparation: Eaten fresh, added to yogurt, oatmeal, or used in baking.

Raspberries

GI: 32

GL: 3 (per 80g portion)

Preparation: Eaten fresh, added to desserts, salads, or made into sauces.

Blackberries

GI: 25

GL: 3 (per 80g portion)

Preparation: Eaten fresh, added to cereals, smoothies, or used in baking.

Cranberries

GI: 45

GL: 2 (per 80g portion)

Preparation: Often consumed dried or in juice, used in sauces or baked goods.

Goji Berries

GI: 29

GL: 4 (per 80g portion)

Preparation: Eaten dried as a snack, added to trail mixes or smoothies.

Cherries

GI: 20

GL: 3 (per 80g portion)

Preparation: Eaten fresh, used in desserts, salads, or made into preserves.

Currants (Black/Red)

GI: 30

GL: 3 (per 80g portion)

Preparation: Eaten fresh, used in jams, jellies, or added to baked goods.

Mulberries

GI: 25

GL: 4 (per 80g portion)

Preparation: Eaten fresh, used in smoothies, salads, or as toppings for desserts.

Elderberries

GI: 35

GL: 4 (per 80g portion)

Preparation: Often used in jams, syrups, or added to baked goods.

Boysenberries

GI: 35

GL: 4 (per 80g portion)

Preparation: Eaten fresh, used in desserts, smoothies, or as toppings.

Huckleberries

GI: 35

GL: 3 (per 80g portion)

Preparation: Eaten fresh, used in jams, pies, or as toppings for yogurt.

Marionberries

GI: 35

GL: 4 (per 80g portion)

Preparation: Eaten fresh, used in baked goods, smoothies, or as toppings.

Loganberries

GI: 35

GL: 4 (per 80g portion)

Preparation: Eaten fresh, used in jams, desserts, or added to yogurt.

Strawberry Guava

GI: 35

GL: 4 (per 80g portion)

Preparation: Eaten fresh, used in fruit salads, or made into jams.

Salmonberries

GI: 35

GL: 4 (per 80g portion)

Preparation: Eaten fresh, used in desserts, or made into jams.

Cloudberries

GI: 35

GL: 4 (per 80g portion)

Preparation: Eaten fresh, used in jams, preserves, or as toppings.

Aronia Berries

GI: 35

GL: 4 (per 80g portion)

Preparation: Eaten fresh, used in juices, smoothies, or as toppings.

Saskatoon Berries

GI: 35

GL: 4 (per 80g portion)

Preparation: Eaten fresh, used in pies, jams, or as toppings.

Serviceberries

GI: 35

GL: 4 (per 80g portion)

Preparation: Eaten fresh, used in desserts, jams, or as toppings.

Juneberries

GI: 35

GL: 4 (per 80g portion)

Preparation: Eaten fresh, used in baking, jams, or as toppings.

Wintergreen Berries

GI: 35

GL: 4 (per 80g portion)

Preparation: Eaten fresh, used in jams, jellies, or as flavorings.

Bilberries

GI: 35

GL: 4 (per 80g portion)

Preparation: Eaten fresh, used in baked goods, jams, or as toppings.

Hackberries

GI: 35

GL: 4 (per 80g portion)

Preparation: Eaten fresh, used in jams, jellies, or as toppings.

Serviceberries

GI: 35

GL: 4 (per 80g portion)

Preparation: Eaten fresh, used in desserts, jams, or as toppings.

Buffaloberries

GI: 35

GL: 4 (per 80g portion)

Preparation: Eaten fresh, used in jams, sauces, or as toppings.

Crowberries

GI: 35

GL: 4 (per 80g portion)

Preparation: Eaten fresh, used in jams, sauces, or as toppings.

Grapeberries

GI: 35

GL: 4 (per 80g portion)

Preparation: Eaten fresh, used in salads, or as toppings.

Chokeberries (Aronia)

GI: 35

GL: 4 (per 80g portion)

Preparation: Eaten fresh, used in juices, smoothies, or as toppings.

Bearberries

GI: 35

GL: 4 (per 80g portion)

Preparation: Eaten fresh, used in jams, sauces, or as toppings.

Citrus Fruits

Grapefruit

GI: 25

GL: 3 (per 120g portion)

Preparation: Sliced and eaten fresh, added to salads, or juiced.

Oranges

GI: 40

GL: 5 (per 120g portion)

Preparation: Peeled and eaten fresh, juiced, or used in fruit salads.

Lemons

GI: 20

GL: 1 (per 120g portion)

Preparation: Squeezed for juice, used as a flavor enhancer in dishes or beverages.

Limes

GI: 20

GL: 1 (per 120g portion)

Preparation: Squeezed for juice, used in beverages, or as a garnish.

Tangerines

GI: 40

GL: 5 (per 120g portion)

Preparation: Peeled and eaten fresh, added to salads, or juiced.

Clementines

GI: 40

GL: 4 (per 120g portion)

Preparation: Peeled and eaten fresh, added to fruit salads or smoothies.

Mandarins

GI: 40

GL: 4 (per 120g portion)

Preparation: Peeled and eaten fresh, added to salads or used in desserts.

Pomelos

GI: 30

GL: 3 (per 120g portion)

Preparation: Sliced and eaten fresh, added to salads, or juiced.

Satsumas

GI: 40

GL: 4 (per 120g portion)

Preparation: Peeled and eaten fresh, added to fruit salads or juiced.

Blood Oranges

GI: 40

GL: 5 (per 120g portion)

Preparation: Sliced and eaten fresh, used in salads, or juiced.

Kumquats

GI: 40

GL: 4 (per 120g portion)

Preparation: Eaten whole, sliced and added to salads, or used in preserves.

Ugli Fruit

GI: 45

GL: 4 (per 120g portion)

Preparation: Sliced and eaten fresh, added to fruit salads or used in smoothies.

Yuzu

GI: 40

GL: 4 (per 120g portion)

Preparation: Juice used in sauces, dressings, or added to beverages.

Citron

GI: 30

GL: 2 (per 120g portion)

Preparation: Zest used in baking, candied peel, or added to beverages.

Bergamot

GI: 40

GL: 4 (per 120g portion)

Preparation: Zest used in flavoring, juice added to beverages or used in desserts.

Seville Oranges

GI: 40

GL: 5 (per 120g portion)

Preparation: Juice used in marmalades, sauces, or as a flavoring agent.

Bitter Oranges

GI: 40

GL: 5 (per 120g portion)

Preparation: Zest used in flavoring, juice used in marinades or dressings.

Tangelo

GI: 40

GL: 4 (per 120g portion)

Preparation: Peeled and eaten fresh, added to fruit salads or used in smoothies.

Calamondin

GI: 40

GL: 4 (per 120g portion)

Preparation: Used in preserves, squeezed for juice, or added to beverages.

Lemonade Fruit

GI: 40

GL: 4 (per 120g portion)

Preparation: Sliced and eaten fresh, added to fruit salads or used in beverages.

Kaffir Lime

GI: 20

GL: 1 (per 120g portion)

Preparation: Leaves used in cooking, zest used for flavoring dishes.

Etrog

GI: 40

GL: 4 (per 120g portion)

Preparation: Peeled and eaten fresh, used in religious ceremonies.

Buddha's Hand

GI: 40

GL: 4 (per 120g portion)

Preparation: Zest used in baking, candied peel, or used as a fragrant decoration.

Australian Finger Lime

GI: 40

GL: 4 (per 120g portion)

Preparation: Pearls used as a garnish, added to dishes or beverages.

Australian Round Lime

GI: 40

GL: 4 (per 120g portion)

Preparation: Sliced and eaten fresh, used in fruit salads or as a garnish.

Australian Desert Lime

GI: 40

GL: 4 (per 120g portion)

Preparation: Used in preserves, squeezed for juice, or added to beverages.

Australian Blood Lime

GI: 40

GL: 4 (per 120g portion)

Preparation: Sliced and eaten fresh, used in fruit salads or as a garnish.

Kabosu

GI: 40

GL: 4 (per 120g portion)

Preparation: Sliced and eaten fresh, used in salads or added to beverages.

Yuzuquat

GI: 40

GL: 4 (per 120g portion)

Preparation: Eaten fresh, used in preserves or added to fruit salads.

Citrange

GI: 40

GL: 4 (per 120g portion)

Preparation: Juice used in beverages or as a flavoring agent in recipes.

Peaches

GI: 42

GL: 5 (per 120g portion)

Preparation: Eaten fresh, grilled, added to salads, or used in desserts.

Plums

GI: 40

GL: 4 (per 120g portion)

Preparation: Eaten fresh, used in jams, baked goods, or poached.

Apricots

GI: 34

GL: 3 (per 120g portion)

Preparation: Eaten fresh, grilled, added to yogurt, or used in baking.

Nectarines

GI: 43

GL: 5 (per 120g portion)

Preparation: Eaten fresh, added to fruit salads, grilled, or used in smoothies.

Cherries

GI: 20

GL: 3 (per 120g portion)

Preparation: Eaten fresh, added to desserts, used in jams, or baked into pies.

Mangoes

GI: 51

GL: 8 (per 120g portion)

Preparation: Eaten fresh, blended into smoothies, added to salads, or used in salsas.

Pluots

GI: 40

GL: 4 (per 120g portion)

Preparation: Eaten fresh, used in desserts, or added to fruit salads.

Pineapple

GI: 51

GL: 6 (per 120g portion)

Preparation: Eaten fresh, grilled, added to fruit salads, or used in smoothies.

Apriums

GI: 34

GL: 3 (per 120g portion)

Preparation: Eaten fresh, used in baking, or added to yogurt.

Pluerry

GI: 40

GL: 4 (per 120g portion)

Preparation: Eaten fresh, used in desserts, or added to fruit salads.

White Peaches

GI: 42

GL: 5 (per 120g portion)

Preparation: Eaten fresh, grilled, added to salads, or used in desserts.

Rainier Cherries

GI: 20

GL: 3 (per 120g portion)

Preparation: Eaten fresh, added to desserts, used in jams, or baked into pies.

Black Plums

GI: 40

GL: 4 (per 120g portion)

Preparation: Eaten fresh, used in jams, baked goods, or poached.

Yellow Nectarines

GI: 43

GL: 5 (per 120g portion)

Preparation: Eaten fresh, added to fruit salads, grilled, or used in smoothies.

Santa Rosa Plums

GI: 40

GL: 4 (per 120g portion)

Preparation: Eaten fresh, used in jams, baked goods, or poached.

Honey Mangoes

GI: 51

GL: 8 (per 120g portion)

Preparation: Eaten fresh, blended into smoothies, added to salads, or used in salsas.

Red Cherries

GI: 20

GL: 3 (per 120g portion)

Preparation: Eaten fresh, added to desserts, used in jams, or baked into pies.

Golden Plums

GI: 40

GL: 4 (per 120g portion)

Preparation: Eaten fresh, used in jams, baked goods, or poached.

Saturn Peaches

GI: 42

GL: 5 (per 120g portion)

Preparation: Eaten fresh, grilled, added to salads, or used in desserts.

Sour Cherries

GI: 20

GL: 3 (per 120g portion)

Preparation: Eaten fresh, added to desserts, used in jams, or baked into pies.

Black Apricots

GI: 34

GL: 3 (per 120g portion)

Preparation: Eaten fresh, used in baking, or added to yogurt.

Flat Peaches

GI: 42

GL: 5 (per 120g portion)

Preparation: Eaten fresh, grilled, added to salads, or used in desserts.

Sapote

GI: 35

GL: 4 (per 120g portion)

Preparation: Eaten fresh, used in smoothies, or added to desserts.

Mirabelle Plums

GI: 40

GL: 4 (per 120g portion)

Preparation: Eaten fresh, used in jams, baked goods, or poached.

Indian Mangoes

GI: 51

GL: 8 (per 120g portion)

Preparation: Eaten fresh, blended into smoothies, added to salads, or used in salsas.

Donut Peaches

GI: 42

GL: 5 (per 120g portion)

Preparation: Eaten fresh, grilled, added to salads, or used in desserts.

Victoria Plums

GI: 40

GL: 4 (per 120g portion)

Preparation: Eaten fresh, used in jams, baked goods, or poached.

Canary Melon

GI: 65

GL: 6 (per 120g portion)

Preparation: Eaten fresh, added to fruit salads, or used in smoothies.

Charentais Melon

GI: 60

GL: 6 (per 120g portion)

Preparation: Eaten fresh, used in fruit salads, or served with prosciutto.

Peachcots

GI: 42

GL: 5 (per 120g portion)

Preparation: Eaten fresh, grilled, added to salads, or used in desserts.

Apples

Granny Smith Apples

GI: 38

GL: 6 (per 120g portion)

Preparation: Eaten fresh, sliced for salads, or used in baking pies and tarts.

Red Delicious Apples

GI: 40

GL: 6 (per 120g portion)

Preparation: Eaten fresh, sliced for snacks, or used in salads.

Golden Delicious Apples

GI: 39

GL: 6 (per 120g portion)

Preparation: Eaten fresh, sliced for snacks, or used in baking and applesauce.

Fuji Apples

GI: 38

GL: 6 (per 120g portion)

Preparation: Eaten fresh, sliced for snacks, or used in fruit salads.

Pink Lady Apples

GI: 40

GL: 6 (per 120g portion)

Preparation: Eaten fresh, sliced for snacks, or used in salads and baking.

Gala Apples

GI: 38

GL: 6 (per 120g portion)

Preparation: Eaten fresh, sliced for snacks, or used in fruit salads.

Honeycrisp Apples

GI: 52

GL: 9 (per 120g portion)

Preparation: Eaten fresh, sliced for snacks, or used in salads and desserts.

Braeburn Apples

GI: 35

GL: 6 (per 120g portion)

Preparation: Eaten fresh, sliced for snacks, or used in baking and salads.

Cripps Pink Apples (Pink Lady variation)

GI: 40

GL: 6 (per 120g portion)

Preparation: Eaten fresh, sliced for snacks, or used in salads and baking.

Ambrosia Apples

GI: 38

GL: 6 (per 120g portion)

Preparation: Eaten fresh, sliced for snacks, or used in fruit salads.

Empire Apples

GI: 40

GL: 6 (per 120g portion)

Preparation: Eaten fresh, sliced for snacks, or used in salads.

Jonagold Apples

GI: 40

GL: 6 (per 120g portion)

Preparation: Eaten fresh, sliced for snacks, or used in baking and salads.

McIntosh Apples

GI: 55

GL: 8 (per 120g portion)

Preparation: Eaten fresh, sliced for snacks, or used in applesauce.

Gravenstein Apples

GI: 40

GL: 6 (per 120g portion)

Preparation: Eaten fresh, sliced for snacks, or used in baking and sauces.

Opal Apples

GI: 36

GL: 6 (per 120g portion)

Preparation: Eaten fresh, sliced for snacks, or used in fruit salads.

Jazz Apples

GI: 42

GL: 6 (per 120g portion)

Preparation: Eaten fresh, sliced for snacks, or used in salads and baking.

Braeburn

GI: 35

GL: 6 (per 120g portion)

Preparation: Eaten fresh, sliced for snacks, or used in baking and salads.

Kanzi Apples

GI: 38

GL: 6 (per 120g portion)

Preparation: Eaten fresh, sliced for snacks, or used in fruit salads.

Pacific Rose Apples

GI: 42

GL: 6 (per 120g portion)

Preparation: Eaten fresh, sliced for snacks, or used in salads and baking.

Envy Apples

GI: 39

GL: 6 (per 120g portion)

Preparation: Eaten fresh, sliced for snacks, or used in fruit salads.

SweeTango Apples

GI: 38

GL: 6 (per 120g portion)

Preparation: Eaten fresh, sliced for snacks, or used in fruit salads.

Eve Apples

GI: 38

GL: 6 (per 120g portion)

Preparation: Eaten fresh, sliced for snacks, or used in baking and salads.

Arkansas Black Apples

GI: 40

GL: 6 (per 120g portion)

Preparation: Eaten fresh, sliced for snacks, or used in baking and salads.

Northern Spy Apples

GI: 58

GL: 9 (per 120g portion)

Preparation: Eaten fresh, sliced for snacks, or used in baking and applesauce.

Cameo Apples

GI: 38

GL: 6 (per 120g portion)

Preparation: Eaten fresh, sliced for snacks, or used in salads and baking.

Akane Apples

GI: 38

GL: 6 (per 120g portion)

Preparation: Eaten fresh, sliced for snacks, or used in fruit salads.

Red Rome Apples

GI: 40

GL: 6 (per 120g portion)

Preparation: Eaten fresh, sliced for snacks, or used in baking and sauces.

Ashmead's Kernel Apples

GI: 40

GL: 6 (per 120g portion)

Preparation: Eaten fresh, sliced for snacks, or used in baking and salads.

Belle de Boskoop Apples

GI: 35

GL: 6 (per 120g portion)

Preparation: Eaten fresh, sliced for snacks, or used in baking and pies.

Roxbury Russet Apples

GI: 38

GL: 6 (per 120g portion)

Preparation: Eaten fresh, sliced for snacks, or used in baking and salads.

Pears

Anjou Pears

GI: 38

GL: 4 (per 120g portion)

Preparation: Eaten fresh, sliced for snacks, used in salads, or baked in desserts.

Bartlett Pears

GI: 41

GL: 5 (per 120g portion)

Preparation: Eaten fresh, sliced for snacks, used in fruit salads, or poached.

Bosc Pears

GI: 38

GL: 4 (per 120g portion)

Preparation: Eaten fresh, sliced for snacks, used in salads, or baked in desserts.

Comice Pears

GI: 38

GL: 4 (per 120g portion)

Preparation: Eaten fresh, sliced for snacks, used in fruit salads, or paired with cheese.

Forelle Pears

GI: 38

GL: 4 (per 120g portion)

Preparation: Eaten fresh, sliced for snacks, used in fruit salads, or poached.

Seckel Pears

GI: 41

GL: 5 (per 120g portion)

Preparation: Eaten fresh, sliced for snacks, used in fruit salads, or pickled.

Starkrimson Pears

GI: 41

GL: 5 (per 120g portion)

Preparation: Eaten fresh, sliced for snacks, used in fruit salads, or paired with cheese.

Concorde Pears

GI: 38

GL: 4 (per 120g portion)

Preparation: Eaten fresh, sliced for snacks, used in salads, or baked in desserts.

Taylor's Gold Pears

GI: 41

GL: 5 (per 120g portion)

Preparation: Eaten fresh, sliced for snacks, used in salads, or poached.

Red Anjou Pears

GI: 38

GL: 4 (per 120g portion)

Preparation: Eaten fresh, sliced for snacks, used in salads, or baked in desserts.

Green Anjou Pears

GI: 38

GL: 4 (per 120g portion)

Preparation: Eaten fresh, sliced for snacks, used in salads, or baked in desserts.

Asian Pears

GI: 25

GL: 3 (per 120g portion)

Preparation: Eaten fresh, sliced for snacks, used in salads, or added to stir-fries.

Red Bartlett Pears

GI: 41

GL: 5 (per 120g portion)

Preparation: Eaten fresh, sliced for snacks, used in fruit salads, or poached.

Golden Russet Pears

GI: 41

GL: 5 (per 120g portion)

Preparation: Eaten fresh, sliced for snacks, used in fruit salads, or baked.

Harrow Delight Pears

GI: 38

GL: 4 (per 120g portion)

Preparation: Eaten fresh, sliced for snacks, used in salads, or baked in desserts.

Harrow Sweet Pears

GI: 38

GL: 4 (per 120g portion)

Preparation: Eaten fresh, sliced for snacks, used in salads, or baked in desserts.

Hosui Pears

GI: 38

GL: 4 (per 120g portion)

Preparation: Eaten fresh, sliced for snacks, used in salads, or poached.

Kieffer Pears

GI: 41

GL: 5 (per 120g portion)

Preparation: Eaten fresh, sliced for snacks, used in fruit salads, or baked.

Moonglow Pears

GI: 38

GL: 4 (per 120g portion)

Preparation: Eaten fresh, sliced for snacks, used in salads, or baked in desserts.

Olympic Pears

GI: 38

GL: 4 (per 120g portion)

Preparation: Eaten fresh, sliced for snacks, used in salads, or baked in desserts.

Passe Crassane Pears

GI: 41

GL: 5 (per 120g portion)

Preparation: Eaten fresh, sliced for snacks, used in fruit salads, or poached.

Red D'Anjou Pears

GI: 38

GL: 4 (per 120g portion)

Preparation: Eaten fresh, sliced for snacks, used in salads, or baked in desserts.

Red Sensation Pears

GI: 38

GL: 4 (per 120g portion)

Preparation: Eaten fresh, sliced for snacks, used in salads, or baked in desserts.

Shenandoah Pears

GI: 41

GL: 5 (per 120g portion)

Preparation: Eaten fresh, sliced for snacks, used in fruit salads, or poached.

Starking Pears

GI: 38

GL: 4 (per 120g portion)

Preparation: Eaten fresh, sliced for snacks, used in salads, or baked in desserts.

Summercrisp Pears

GI: 41

GL: 5 (per 120g portion)

Preparation: Eaten fresh, sliced for snacks, used in fruit salads, or baked.

Tosca Pears

GI: 38

GL: 4 (per 120g portion)

Preparation: Eaten fresh, sliced for snacks, used in salads, or baked in desserts.

Warren Pears

GI: 38

GL: 4 (per 120g portion)

Preparation: Eaten fresh, sliced for snacks, used in salads, or baked in desserts.

Yali Pears

GI: 41

GL: 5 (per 120g portion)

Preparation: Eaten fresh, sliced for snacks, used in fruit salads, or poached.

Winter Nelis Pears

GI: 41

GL: 5 (per 120g portion)

Preparation: Eaten fresh, sliced for snacks, used in fruit salads, or baked.

Cherries

Bing Cherries

GI: 22

GL: 3 (per 120g portion)

Preparation: Eaten fresh, used in desserts, added to salads, or as a topping.

Rainier Cherries

GI: 22

GL: 3 (per 120g portion)

Preparation: Eaten fresh, used in desserts, added to salads, or enjoyed as a snack.

Sweetheart Cherries

GI: 22

GL: 3 (per 120g portion)

Preparation: Eaten fresh, used in desserts, added to salads, or paired with cheese.

Lapins Cherries

GI: 22

GL: 3 (per 120g portion)

Preparation: Eaten fresh, used in desserts, added to salads, or enjoyed as a snack.

Stella Cherries

GI: 22

GL: 3 (per 120g portion)

Preparation: Eaten fresh, used in desserts, added to salads, or enjoyed as a snack.

Skeena Cherries

GI: 22

GL: 3 (per 120g portion)

Preparation: Eaten fresh, used in desserts, added to salads, or enjoyed as a snack.

Santina Cherries

GI: 22

GL: 3 (per 120g portion)

Preparation: Eaten fresh, used in desserts, added to salads, or enjoyed as a snack.

Tieton Cherries

GI: 22

GL: 3 (per 120g portion)

Preparation: Eaten fresh, used in desserts, added to salads, or enjoyed as a snack.

Regina Cherries

GI: 22

GL: 3 (per 120g portion)

Preparation: Eaten fresh, used in desserts, added to salads, or enjoyed as a snack.

Attika Cherries

GI: 22

GL: 3 (per 120g portion)

Preparation: Eaten fresh, used in desserts, added to salads, or enjoyed as a snack.

Brooks Cherries

GI: 22

GL: 3 (per 120g portion)

Preparation: Eaten fresh, used in desserts, added to salads, or enjoyed as a snack.

Hedelfingen Cherries

GI: 22

GL: 3 (per 120g portion)

Preparation: Eaten fresh, used in desserts, added to salads, or enjoyed as a snack.

Emperor Francis Cherries

GI: 22

GL: 3 (per 120g portion)

Preparation: Eaten fresh, used in desserts, added to salads, or enjoyed as a snack.

Gold Cherry

GI: 22

GL: 3 (per 120g portion)

Preparation: Eaten fresh, used in desserts, added to salads, or enjoyed as a snack.

Hudson Cherries

GI: 22

GL: 3 (per 120g portion)

Preparation: Eaten fresh, used in desserts, added to salads, or enjoyed as a snack.

Kordia Cherries

GI: 22

GL: 3 (per 120g portion)

Preparation: Eaten fresh, used in desserts, added to salads, or enjoyed as a snack.

Larian Cherries

GI: 22

GL: 3 (per 120g portion)

Preparation: Eaten fresh, used in desserts, added to salads, or enjoyed as a snack.

Merton Glory Cherries

GI: 22

GL: 3 (per 120g portion)

Preparation: Eaten fresh, used in desserts, added to salads, or enjoyed as a snack.

Merton Premier Cherries

GI: 22

GL: 3 (per 120g portion)

Preparation: Eaten fresh, used in desserts, added to salads, or enjoyed as a snack.

Sylvia Cherries

GI: 22

GL: 3 (per 120g portion)

Preparation: Eaten fresh, used in desserts, added to salads, or enjoyed as a snack.

Utah Giant Cherries

GI: 22

GL: 3 (per 120g portion)

Preparation: Eaten fresh, used in desserts, added to salads, or enjoyed as a snack.

Vic Cherries

GI: 22

GL: 3 (per 120g portion)

Preparation: Eaten fresh, used in desserts, added to salads, or enjoyed as a snack.

White Gold Cherries

GI: 22

GL: 3 (per 120g portion)

Preparation: Eaten fresh, used in desserts, added to salads, or enjoyed as a snack.

Blushing Gold Cherries

GI: 22

GL: 3 (per 120g portion)

Preparation: Eaten fresh, used in desserts, added to salads, or enjoyed as a snack.

Early Rivers Cherries

GI: 22

GL: 3 (per 120g portion)

Preparation: Eaten fresh, used in desserts, added to salads, or enjoyed as a snack.

Edinburgh Cherries

GI: 22

GL: 3 (per 120g portion)

Preparation: Eaten fresh, used in desserts, added to salads, or enjoyed as a snack.

Goodland Cherries

GI: 22

GL: 3 (per 120g portion)

Preparation: Eaten fresh, used in desserts, added to salads, or enjoyed as a snack.

Helen Cherries

GI: 22

GL: 3 (per 120g portion)

Preparation: Eaten fresh, used in desserts, added to salads, or enjoyed as a snack.

Jeff Cherries

GI: 22

GL: 3 (per 120g portion)

Preparation: Eaten fresh, used in desserts, added to salads, or enjoyed as a snack.

Lambert Cherries

GI: 22

GL: 3 (per 120g portion)

Preparation: Eaten fresh, used in desserts, added to salads, or enjoyed as a snack.

Apricots

Moorpark Apricots

GI: 34

GL: 4 (per 120g portion)

Preparation: Eaten fresh, sliced for snacks, used in salads, or baked in desserts.

Goldcot Apricots

GI: 34

GL: 4 (per 120g portion)

Preparation: Eaten fresh, sliced for snacks, used in jams, or added to yogurt.

Tilton Apricots

GI: 34

GL: 4 (per 120g portion)

Preparation: Eaten fresh, sliced for snacks, used in preserves, or baked in pastries.

Blenheim Apricots

GI: 34

GL: 4 (per 120g portion)

Preparation: Eaten fresh, sliced for snacks, used in jams, or baked in desserts.

Royal Apricots

GI: 34

GL: 4 (per 120g portion)

Preparation: Eaten fresh, sliced for snacks, used in compotes, or added to smoothies.

Harcot Apricots

GI: 34

GL: 4 (per 120g portion)

Preparation: Eaten fresh, sliced for snacks, used in chutneys, or baked in pies.

Autumn Glo Apricots

GI: 34

GL: 4 (per 120g portion)

Preparation: Eaten fresh, sliced for snacks, used in sauces, or added to fruit salads.

Goldbar Apricots

GI: 34

GL: 4 (per 120g portion)

Preparation: Eaten fresh, sliced for snacks, used in jams, or baked in pastries.

Flavor Delight Apricots

GI: 34

GL: 4 (per 120g portion)

Preparation: Eaten fresh, sliced for snacks, used in compotes, or added to yogurt.

Harglow Apricots

GI: 34

GL: 4 (per 120g portion)

Preparation: Eaten fresh, sliced for snacks, used in preserves, or baked in desserts.

Katy Apricots

GI: 34

GL: 4 (per 120g portion)

Preparation: Eaten fresh, sliced for snacks, used in jams, or added to yogurt.

Lorna Apricots

GI: 34

GL: 4 (per 120g portion)

Preparation: Eaten fresh, sliced for snacks, used in chutneys, or baked in pies.

Moorpark Apricots

GI: 34

GL: 4 (per 120g portion)

Preparation: Eaten fresh, sliced for snacks, used in compotes, or added to fruit salads.

Perfection Apricots

GI: 34

GL: 4 (per 120g portion)

Preparation: Eaten fresh, sliced for snacks, used in sauces, or baked in pastries.

Rival Apricots

GI: 34

GL: 4 (per 120g portion)

Preparation: Eaten fresh, sliced for snacks, used in jams, or added to yogurt.

Skaha Apricots

GI: 34

GL: 4 (per 120g portion)

Preparation: Eaten fresh, sliced for snacks, used in chutneys, or baked in pies.

Tomcot Apricots

GI: 34

GL: 4 (per 120g portion)

Preparation: Eaten fresh, sliced for snacks, used in compotes, or added to fruit salads.

Zard Apricots

GI: 34

GL: 4 (per 120g portion)

Preparation: Eaten fresh, sliced for snacks, used in sauces, or baked in pastries.

Flavor Delight Aprium

GI: 34

GL: 4 (per 120g portion)

Preparation: Eaten fresh, sliced for snacks, used in compotes, or added to yogurt.

Goldrich Apricots

GI: 34

GL: 4 (per 120g portion)

Preparation: Eaten fresh, sliced for snacks, used in chutneys, or baked in pies.

Goldstrike Apricots

GI: 34

GL: 4 (per 120g portion)

Preparation: Eaten fresh, sliced for snacks, used in jams, or added to yogurt.

Leah Cot Apricots

GI: 34

GL: 4 (per 120g portion)

Preparation: Eaten fresh, sliced for snacks, used in sauces, or baked in pastries.

Pixie Cot Apricots

GI: 34

GL: 4 (per 120g portion)

Preparation: Eaten fresh, sliced for snacks, used in compotes, or added to fruit salads.

Primadonna Apricots

GI: 34

GL: 4 (per 120g portion)

Preparation: Eaten fresh, sliced for snacks, used in chutneys, or baked in pies.

Rival Apricots

GI: 34

GL: 4 (per 120g portion)

Preparation: Eaten fresh, sliced for snacks, used in jams, or added to yogurt.

Spring Blush Apricots

GI: 34

GL: 4 (per 120g portion)

Preparation: Eaten fresh, sliced for snacks, used in sauces, or baked in pastries.

Sunglo Apricots

GI: 34

GL: 4 (per 120g portion)

Preparation: Eaten fresh, sliced for snacks, used in compotes, or added to fruit salads.

Tilton Apricots

GI: 34

GL: 4 (per 120g portion)

Preparation: Eaten fresh, sliced for snacks, used in chutneys, or baked in pies.

Vergers Apricots

GI: 34

GL: 4 (per 120g portion)

Preparation: Eaten fresh, sliced for snacks, used in jams, or added to yogurt.

Vivagold Apricots

GI: 34

GL: 4 (per 120g portion)

Preparation: Eaten fresh, sliced for snacks, used in sauces, or baked in pastries.

Varieties of Grapes

Red Seedless Grapes

GI: 43

GL: 5 (per 120g portion)

Preparation: Eaten fresh as a snack, added to salads, or frozen for a refreshing treat.

Green Seedless Grapes

GI: 43

GL: 5 (per 120g portion)

Preparation: Eaten fresh as a snack, used in fruit salads, or paired with cheese.

Black Seedless Grapes

GI: 43

GL: 5 (per 120g portion)

Preparation: Eaten fresh as a snack, used in desserts, or blended into smoothies.

Concord Grapes

GI: 53

GL: 6 (per 120g portion)

Preparation: Eaten fresh as a snack, used in jams, or made into grape juice.

Cotton Candy Grapes

GI: 43

GL: 5 (per 120g portion)

Preparation: Eaten fresh as a snack, used in fruit salads, or frozen for a sweet treat.

Muscat Grapes

GI: 43

GL: 5 (per 120g portion)

Preparation: Eaten fresh as a snack, used in desserts, or added to cheese platters.

Flame Seedless Grapes

GI: 43

GL: 5 (per 120g portion)

Preparation: Eaten fresh as a snack, used in fruit salads, or added to yogurt.

Thompson Seedless Grapes

GI: 43

GL: 5 (per 120g portion)

Preparation: Eaten fresh as a snack, used in desserts, or frozen for a cool treat.

Ruby Roman Grapes

GI: 43

GL: 5 (per 120g portion)

Preparation: Eaten fresh as a premium snack, used in desserts, or added to wine.

Muscadine Grapes

GI: 53

GL: 6 (per 120g portion)

Preparation: Eaten fresh as a snack, used in jams, or made into wine.

Niagara Grapes

GI: 43

GL: 5 (per 120g portion)

Preparation: Eaten fresh as a snack, used in desserts, or juiced for beverages.

Perlette Grapes

GI: 43

GL: 5 (per 120g portion)

Preparation: Eaten fresh as a snack, used in fruit salads, or added to cheese platters.

Riesling Grapes

GI: 43

GL: 5 (per 120g portion)

Preparation: Eaten fresh as a snack, used in desserts, or juiced for beverages.

Sultana Grapes

GI: 43

GL: 5 (per 120g portion)

Preparation: Eaten fresh as a snack, used in baking, or added to trail mixes.

Zante Currant Grapes

GI: 43

GL: 5 (per 120g portion)

Preparation: Eaten fresh as a snack, used in baking, or added to oatmeal.

Autumn Royal Grapes

GI: 43

GL: 5 (per 120g portion)

Preparation: Eaten fresh as a snack, used in fruit salads, or frozen for a refreshing treat.

Champagne Grapes

GI: 43

GL: 5 (per 120g portion)

Preparation: Eaten fresh as a snack, used in desserts, or added to cheese platters.

Crimson Seedless Grapes

GI: 43

GL: 5 (per 120g portion)

Preparation: Eaten fresh as a snack, used in fruit salads, or frozen for a cool treat.

Kyoho Grapes

GI: 43

GL: 5 (per 120g portion)

Preparation: Eaten fresh as a snack, used in desserts, or juiced for beverages.

Reliance Grapes

GI: 43

GL: 5 (per 120g portion)

Preparation: Eaten fresh as a snack, used in fruit salads, or added to yogurt.

Ruby Cabernet Grapes

GI: 43

GL: 5 (per 120g portion)

Preparation: Eaten fresh as a snack, used in desserts, or juiced for beverages.

Black Corinth Grapes

GI: 43

GL: 5 (per 120g portion)

Preparation: Eaten fresh as a snack, used in baking, or added to oatmeal.

Cardinal Grapes

GI: 43

GL: 5 (per 120g portion)

Preparation: Eaten fresh as a snack, used in fruit salads, or frozen for a refreshing treat.

Fantasy Grapes

GI: 43

GL: 5 (per 120g portion)

Preparation: Eaten fresh as a snack, used in desserts, or added to cheese platters.

Himrod Grapes

GI: 43

GL: 5 (per 120g portion)

Preparation: Eaten fresh as a snack, used in fruit salads, or frozen for a cool treat.

Italia Grapes

GI: 43

GL: 5 (per 120g portion)

Preparation: Eaten fresh as a snack, used in desserts, or juiced for beverages.

Moon Drop Grapes

GI: 43

GL: 5 (per 120g portion)

Preparation: Eaten fresh as a snack, used in fruit salads, or frozen for a refreshing treat.

Pixie Grapes

GI: 43

GL: 5 (per 120g portion)

Preparation: Eaten fresh as a snack, used in desserts, or added to yogurt.

Rish Baba Grapes

GI: 43

GL: 5 (per 120g portion)

Preparation: Eaten fresh as a snack, used in jams, or made into grape juice.

Suffolk Red Grapes

GI: 43

GL: 5 (per 120g portion)

Preparation: Eaten fresh as a snack, used in fruit salads, or added to cheese platters.

Varieties of Kiwi

Green Kiwifruit

GI: 39

GL: 5 (per 120g portion)

Preparation: Peeled and eaten fresh, sliced for snacks, added to fruit salads, or blended into smoothies.

Gold Kiwifruit

GI: 38

GL: 6 (per 120g portion)

Preparation: Peeled and eaten fresh, sliced for snacks, added to yogurt, or used in desserts.

Baby Kiwi (Hardy Kiwi)

GI: 50

GL: 4 (per 120g portion)

Preparation: Eaten whole or sliced, added to salads, used in jams, or enjoyed as a fresh snack.

Red Kiwifruit

GI: 44

GL: 5 (per 120g portion)

Preparation: Peeled and eaten fresh, sliced for snacks, added to fruit salads, or blended into smoothies.

Kiwi Berries

GI: 53

GL: 4 (per 120g portion)

Preparation: Eaten whole or sliced, added to desserts, used in preserves, or enjoyed fresh as a snack.

Arctic Kiwi (Hardy Kiwi)

GI: 53

GL: 5 (per 120g portion)

Preparation: Eaten whole or sliced, added to fruit salads, used in jams, or enjoyed fresh as a snack.

Issai Hardy Kiwi

GI: 58

GL: 4 (per 120g portion)

Preparation: Eaten whole or sliced, added to smoothies, used in desserts, or enjoyed as a fresh snack.

Ananasnaya Hardy Kiwi

GI: 53

GL: 5 (per 120g portion)

Preparation: Eaten whole or sliced, added to fruit salads, used in jams, or enjoyed fresh as a snack.

Tara Hardy Kiwi

GI: 56

GL: 4 (per 120g portion)

Preparation: Eaten whole or sliced, added to salads, used in desserts, or enjoyed as a fresh snack.

Weiki Hardy Kiwi

GI: 54

GL: 5 (per 120g portion)

Preparation: Eaten whole or sliced, added to yogurt, used in jams, or enjoyed fresh as a snack.

Jenny Hardy Kiwi

GI: 54

GL: 5 (per 120g portion)

Preparation: Eaten whole or sliced, added to fruit salads, used in preserves, or enjoyed fresh as a snack.

Ken's Red Hardy Kiwi

GI: 53

GL: 5 (per 120g portion)

Preparation: Eaten whole or sliced, added to smoothies, used in desserts, or enjoyed as a fresh snack.

Vincent Hardy Kiwi

GI: 54

GL: 5 (per 120g portion)

Preparation: Eaten whole or sliced, added to salads, used in jams, or enjoyed fresh as a snack.

MSU (Michigan State University) Hardy Kiwi

GI: 53

GL: 5 (per 120g portion)

Preparation: Eaten whole or sliced, added to fruit salads, used in preserves, or enjoyed fresh as a snack.

Tatyana Hardy Kiwi

GI: 54

GL: 5 (per 120g portion)

Preparation: Eaten whole or sliced, added to yogurt, used in desserts, or enjoyed fresh as a snack.

Eva Hardy Kiwi

GI: 55

GL: 5 (per 120g portion)

Preparation: Eaten whole or sliced, added to smoothies, used in jams, or enjoyed fresh as a snack.

Matua Hardy Kiwi

GI: 54

GL: 5 (per 120g portion)

Preparation: Eaten whole or sliced, added to fruit salads, used in preserves, or enjoyed fresh as a snack.

Krupnopladnaya Hardy Kiwi

GI: 56

GL: 4 (per 120g portion)

Preparation: Eaten whole or sliced, added to salads, used in desserts, or enjoyed fresh as a snack.

Zonguldak Hardy Kiwi

GI: 56

GL: 4 (per 120g portion)

Preparation: Eaten whole or sliced, added to yogurt, used in jams, or enjoyed fresh as a snack.

Leo Hardy Kiwi

GI: 56

GL: 4 (per 120g portion)

Preparation: Eaten whole or sliced, added to smoothies, used in desserts, or enjoyed fresh as a snack.

Saanichton Hardy Kiwi

GI: 55

GL: 5 (per 120g portion)

Preparation: Eaten whole or sliced, added to fruit salads, used in preserves, or enjoyed fresh as a snack.

Hort16A Gold Kiwifruit

GI: 38

GL: 6 (per 120g portion)

Preparation: Peeled and eaten fresh, sliced for snacks, added to yogurt, or used in desserts.

Hayward Green Kiwifruit

GI: 39

GL: 5 (per 120g portion)

Preparation: Peeled and eaten fresh, sliced for snacks, added to fruit salads, or blended into smoothies.

Red Kiwi

GI: 45

GL: 5 (per 120g portion)

Preparation: Peeled and eaten fresh, sliced for snacks, added to fruit salads, or blended into smoothies.

Hardy Red Kiwi

GI: 54

GL: 5 (per 120g portion)

Preparation: Eaten whole or sliced, added to yogurt, used in jams, or enjoyed fresh as a snack.

Kiwi Star

GI: 54

GL: 5 (per 120g portion)

Preparation: Eaten whole or sliced, added to salads, used in desserts, or enjoyed fresh as a snack.

Hardy Anna Kiwi

GI: 55

GL: 5 (per 120g portion)

Preparation: Eaten whole or sliced, added to smoothies, used in jams, or enjoyed fresh as a snack.

Anna Hardy Kiwi

GI: 54

GL: 5 (per 120g portion)

Preparation: Eaten whole or sliced, added to fruit salads, used in preserves, or enjoyed fresh as a snack.

Weiki Kiwi

GI: 56

GL: 4 (per 120g portion)

Preparation: Eaten whole or sliced, added to yogurt, used in jams, or enjoyed fresh as a snack.

Tamu Hardy Kiwi

GI: 55

GL: 5 (per 120g portion)

Preparation: Eaten whole or sliced, added to smoothies, used in desserts, or enjoyed fresh as a snack.

Varieties of Oranges

Navel Oranges

GI: 40

GL: 5 (per medium-sized orange)

Portion Size: 1 medium orange

Preparation: Peeled and eaten fresh, juiced for beverages, or used in fruit salads.

Valencia Oranges

GI: 43

GL: 6 (per medium-sized orange)

Portion Size: 1 medium orange

Preparation: Squeezed for fresh orange juice, eaten fresh, or added to fruit salads.

Blood Oranges

GI: 40

GL: 5 (per medium-sized orange)

Portion Size: 1 medium orange

Preparation: Enjoyed fresh, used in salads, or juiced for a distinctive red-orange beverage.

Cara Cara Oranges

GI: 40

GL: 4 (per medium-sized orange)

Portion Size: 1 medium orange

Preparation: Eaten fresh, juiced for beverages, or added to fruit platters.

Seville Oranges

GI: 43

GL: 5 (per medium-sized orange)

Portion Size: 1 medium orange

Preparation: Primarily used for making marmalade or citrus-based sauces.

Mandarin Oranges

GI: 45

GL: 6 (per medium-sized orange)

Portion Size: 1 medium orange

Preparation: Peeled and eaten fresh, used in salads, or canned for convenience.

Satsuma Oranges

GI: 42

GL: 5 (per medium-sized orange)

Portion Size: 1 medium orange

Preparation: Easily peeled and eaten fresh, used in fruit salads, or juiced for beverages.

Tangerines

GI: 42

GL: 6 (per medium-sized orange)

Portion Size: 1 medium orange

Preparation: Peeled and eaten fresh, added to salads, or used in fruit desserts.

Minneola Tangelo

GI: 43

GL: 5 (per medium-sized orange)

Portion Size: 1 medium orange

Preparation: Eaten fresh, juiced for beverages, or added to fruit platters.

Clementines

GI: 35

GL: 4 (per medium-sized orange)

Portion Size: 1 medium orange

Preparation: Easily peeled and eaten fresh, added to salads, or used in desserts.

Temple Oranges

GI: 35

GL: 4 (per medium-sized orange)

Portion Size: 1 medium orange

Preparation: Eaten fresh, juiced for beverages, or used in fruit salads.

Tangor Oranges

GI: 35

GL: 4 (per medium-sized orange)

Portion Size: 1 medium orange

Preparation: Enjoyed fresh, used in salads, or juiced for beverages.

Bergamot Oranges

GI: 40

GL: 5 (per medium-sized orange)

Portion Size: 1 medium orange

Preparation: Primarily used for flavoring in teas, essential oils, or making marmalade.

Kumquats

GI: 40

GL: 4 (per serving - approx. 5 kumquats)

Portion Size: About 5 kumquats

Preparation: Eaten whole (including the peel), used in salads, or preserved in syrups.

Pixie Oranges

GI: 43

GL: 5 (per medium-sized orange)

Portion Size: 1 medium orange

Preparation: Enjoyed fresh, juiced for beverages, or added to fruit platters.

Jaffa Oranges

GI: 43

GL: 5 (per medium-sized orange)

Portion Size: 1 medium orange

Preparation: Eaten fresh, juiced for beverages, or used in fruit salads.

Bitter Orange

GI: 43

GL: 5 (per medium-sized orange)

Portion Size: 1 medium orange

Preparation: Primarily used for making marmalade, candied peel, or in savory dishes.

Tangelo

GI: 43

GL: 5 (per medium-sized orange)

Portion Size: 1 medium orange

Preparation: Enjoyed fresh, juiced for beverages, or added to fruit platters.

Ambersweet Oranges

GI: 43

GL: 5 (per medium-sized orange)

Portion Size: 1 medium orange

Preparation: Eaten fresh, juiced for beverages, or used in fruit salads.

Washington Navel Oranges

GI: 40

GL: 5 (per medium-sized orange)

Portion Size: 1 medium orange

Preparation: Peeled and eaten fresh, juiced for beverages, or used in fruit salads.

Navelina Oranges

GI: 40

GL: 5 (per medium-sized orange)

Portion Size: 1 medium orange

Preparation: Eaten fresh, juiced for beverages, or used in fruit salads.

Hamlin Oranges

GI: 40

GL: 5 (per medium-sized orange)

Portion Size: 1 medium orange

Preparation: Enjoyed fresh, juiced for beverages, or used in fruit salads.

Cara Cara Navels

GI: 40

GL: 4 (per medium-sized orange)

Portion Size: 1 medium orange

Preparation: Peeled and eaten fresh, juiced for beverages, or used in fruit salads.

Seville Sour Oranges

GI: 43

GL: 5 (per medium-sized orange)

Portion Size: 1 medium orange

Preparation: Primarily used for making marmalade or sour orange-based sauces.

Pineapple Oranges

GI: 40

GL: 5 (per medium-sized orange)

Portion Size: 1 medium orange

Preparation: Eaten fresh, juiced for beverages, or used in fruit salads.

Barnfield Navel Oranges

GI: 40

GL: 5 (per medium-sized orange)

Portion Size: 1 medium orange

Preparation: Peeled and eaten fresh, juiced for beverages, or used in fruit salads.

Delta Oranges

GI: 43

GL: 5 (per medium-sized orange)

Portion Size: 1 medium orange

Preparation: Enjoyed fresh, juiced for beverages, or used in fruit salads.

Navelate Oranges

GI: 40

GL: 5 (per medium-sized orange)

Portion Size: 1 medium orange

Preparation: Eaten fresh, juiced for beverages, or used in fruit salads.

Berna Oranges

GI: 43

GL: 5 (per medium-sized orange)

Portion Size: 1 medium orange

Preparation: Enjoyed fresh, juiced for beverages, or used in fruit salads.

Salustiana Oranges

GI: 40

GL: 5 (per medium-sized orange)

Portion Size: 1 medium orange

Preparation: Peeled and eaten fresh, juiced for beverages, or used in fruit salads.

Varieties of Plums

Black Plum (Japanese Plum)

GI: 39

GL: 4 (per medium-sized plum)

Portion Size: 1 medium plum

Preparation: Eaten fresh, added to fruit salads, or used in jams and desserts.

Red Plum

GI: 40

GL: 4 (per medium-sized plum)

Portion Size: 1 medium plum

Preparation: Eaten fresh, used in baked goods, or sliced for snacks.

Yellow Plum

GI: 40

GL: 4 (per medium-sized plum)

Portion Size: 1 medium plum

Preparation: Enjoyed fresh, used in fruit salads, or made into compote.

Green Plum

GI: 39

GL: 4 (per medium-sized plum)

Portion Size: 1 medium plum

Preparation: Eaten fresh, used in pickling, or enjoyed with salt.

Damson Plum

GI: 39

GL: 4 (per medium-sized plum)

Portion Size: 1 medium plum

Preparation: Eaten fresh, used in jams, or made into sauces for savory dishes.

Victoria Plum

GI: 40

GL: 4 (per medium-sized plum)

Portion Size: 1 medium plum

Preparation: Eaten fresh, used in desserts, or made into jams and preserves.

Satsuma Plum

GI: 40

GL: 4 (per medium-sized plum)

Portion Size: 1 medium plum

Preparation: Eaten fresh, used in compotes, or added to savory dishes.

Santa Rosa Plum

GI: 39

GL: 4 (per medium-sized plum)

Portion Size: 1 medium plum

Preparation: Eaten fresh, used in desserts, or made into sauces.

Elephant Heart Plum

GI: 40

GL: 4 (per medium-sized plum)

Portion Size: 1 medium plum

Preparation: Eaten fresh, used in baking, or enjoyed as a snack.

Laroda Plum

GI: 39

GL: 4 (per medium-sized plum)

Portion Size: 1 medium plum

Preparation: Eaten fresh, used in desserts, or made into jams.

Ruby Queen Plum

GI: 40

GL: 4 (per medium-sized plum)

Portion Size: 1 medium plum

Preparation: Eaten fresh, used in salads, or made into sauces.

Friar Plum

GI: 40

GL: 4 (per medium-sized plum)

Portion Size: 1 medium plum

Preparation: Eaten fresh, used in baking, or enjoyed as a snack.

President Plum

GI: 39

GL: 4 (per medium-sized plum)

Portion Size: 1 medium plum

Preparation: Eaten fresh, used in desserts, or made into jams.

Mariposa Plum

GI: 40

GL: 4 (per medium-sized plum)

Portion Size: 1 medium plum

Preparation: Eaten fresh, used in baking, or enjoyed as a snack.

Early Golden Plum

GI: 40

GL: 4 (per medium-sized plum)

Portion Size: 1 medium plum

Preparation: Eaten fresh, used in compotes, or made into jams.

Burbank Plum

GI: 39

GL: 4 (per medium-sized plum)

Portion Size: 1 medium plum

Preparation: Eaten fresh, used in desserts, or made into sauces.

Owen T-3 Plum

GI: 40

GL: 4 (per medium-sized plum)

Portion Size: 1 medium plum

Preparation: Eaten fresh, used in baking, or enjoyed as a snack.

Late Santa Rosa Plum

GI: 39

GL: 4 (per medium-sized plum)

Portion Size: 1 medium plum

Preparation: Eaten fresh, used in desserts, or made into jams.

El Dorado Plum

GI: 40

GL: 4 (per medium-sized plum)

Portion Size: 1 medium plum

Preparation: Eaten fresh, used in baking, or enjoyed as a snack.

Howard Sun Plum

GI: 39

GL: 4 (per medium-sized plum)

Portion Size: 1 medium plum

Preparation: Eaten fresh, used in desserts, or made into sauces.

Methley Plum

GI: 40

GL: 4 (per medium-sized plum)

Portion Size: 1 medium plum

Preparation: Eaten fresh, used in compotes, or made into jams.

Golden Nectar Plum

GI: 40

GL: 4 (per medium-sized plum)

Portion Size: 1 medium plum

Preparation: Eaten fresh, used in baking, or enjoyed as a snack.

Green Gage Plum

GI: 39

GL: 4 (per medium-sized plum)

Portion Size: 1 medium plum

Preparation: Eaten fresh, used in desserts, or made into jams.

Improved French Plum

GI: 40

GL: 4 (per medium-sized plum)

Portion Size: 1 medium plum

Preparation: Eaten fresh, used in compotes, or made into sauces.

Kelsey Plum

GI: 39

GL: 4 (per medium-sized plum)

Portion Size: 1 medium plum

Preparation: Eaten fresh, used in desserts, or made into jams.

Ruby Sweet Plum

GI: 40

GL: 4 (per medium-sized plum)

Portion Size: 1 medium plum

Preparation: Eaten fresh, used in baking, or enjoyed as a snack.

Santa Barbara Plum

GI: 39

GL: 4 (per medium-sized plum)

Portion Size: 1 medium plum

Preparation: Eaten fresh, used in desserts, or made into sauces.

Tokyo Rose Plum

GI: 40

GL: 4 (per medium-sized plum)

Portion Size: 1 medium plum

Preparation: Eaten fresh, used in compotes, or made into jams.

Wickson Plum

GI: 39

GL: 4 (per medium-sized plum)

Portion Size: 1 medium plum

Preparation: Eaten fresh, used in desserts, or made into sauces.

Yellow Egg Plum

GI: 40

GL: 4 (per medium-sized plum)

Portion Size: 1 medium plum

Preparation: Eaten fresh, used in baking, or enjoyed as a snack.

Peaches

Yellow Peach

GI: 42

GL: 5 (per medium-sized peach)

Portion Size: 1 medium peach

Preparation: Eaten fresh, grilled for desserts, or added to salads.

White Peach

GI: 40

GL: 5 (per medium-sized peach)

Portion Size: 1 medium peach

Preparation: Enjoyed fresh, used in fruit salads, or blended into smoothies.

Donut Peach

GI: 42

GL: 4 (per medium-sized peach)

Portion Size: 1 medium peach

Preparation: Eaten fresh, used in baking, or sliced for snacks.

Nectarine

GI: 43

GL: 4 (per medium-sized nectarine)

Portion Size: 1 medium nectarine

Preparation: Eaten fresh, sliced for snacks, or used in desserts.

Flat Peach

GI: 40

GL: 4 (per medium-sized peach)

Portion Size: 1 medium peach

Preparation: Enjoyed fresh, used in fruit salads, or grilled for desserts.

Saturn Peach

GI: 42

GL: 4 (per medium-sized peach)

Portion Size: 1 medium peach

Preparation: Eaten fresh, used in desserts, or added to yogurt.

Red Haven Peach

GI: 41

GL: 5 (per medium-sized peach)

Portion Size: 1 medium peach

Preparation: Enjoyed fresh, used in baking, or sliced for snacks.

Babcock Peach

GI: 40

GL: 5 (per medium-sized peach)

Portion Size: 1 medium peach

Preparation: Eaten fresh, used in fruit salads, or blended into smoothies.

Elberta Peach

GI: 42

GL: 5 (per medium-sized peach)

Portion Size: 1 medium peach

Preparation: Enjoyed fresh, used in desserts, or added to salads.

Glen Glo Peach

GI: 43

GL: 5 (per medium-sized peach)

Portion Size: 1 medium peach

Preparation: Eaten fresh, used in baking, or sliced for snacks.

Fairtime Peach

GI: 41

GL: 5 (per medium-sized peach)

Portion Size: 1 medium peach

Preparation: Enjoyed fresh, used in fruit salads, or grilled for desserts.

June Pride Peach

GI: 40

GL: 5 (per medium-sized peach)

Portion Size: 1 medium peach

Preparation: Eaten fresh, used in desserts, or added to yogurt.

White Lady Peach

GI: 42

GL: 5 (per medium-sized peach)

Portion Size: 1 medium peach

Preparation: Enjoyed fresh, used in baking, or sliced for snacks.

Red Globe Peach

GI: 41

GL: 5 (per medium-sized peach)

Portion Size: 1 medium peach

Preparation: Eaten fresh, used in fruit salads, or blended into smoothies.

Sugar Giant Peach

GI: 40

GL: 5 (per medium-sized peach)

Portion Size: 1 medium peach

Preparation: Enjoyed fresh, used in desserts, or added to salads.

Fay Elberta Peach

GI: 42

GL: 5 (per medium-sized peach)

Portion Size: 1 medium peach

Preparation: Eaten fresh, used in baking, or sliced for snacks.

Snow Giant Peach

GI: 43

GL: 5 (per medium-sized peach)

Portion Size: 1 medium peach

Preparation: Enjoyed fresh, used in fruit salads, or blended into smoothies.

August Pride Peach

GI: 41

GL: 5 (per medium-sized peach)

Portion Size: 1 medium peach

Preparation: Eaten fresh, used in desserts, or added to yogurt.

Golden Jubilee Peach

GI: 40

GL: 5 (per medium-sized peach)

Portion Size: 1 medium peach

Preparation: Enjoyed fresh, used in baking, or sliced for snacks.

Indian Blood Peach

GI: 42

GL: 5 (per medium-sized peach)

Portion Size: 1 medium peach

Preparation: Eaten fresh, used in fruit salads, or blended into smoothies.

Indian Free Peach

GI: 43

GL: 5 (per medium-sized peach)

Portion Size: 1 medium peach

Preparation: Enjoyed fresh, used in desserts, or added to salads.

Red Wing Peach

GI: 41

GL: 5 (per medium-sized peach)

Portion Size: 1 medium peach

Preparation: Eaten fresh, used in baking, or sliced for snacks.

August Giant Peach

GI: 40

GL: 5 (per medium-sized peach)

Portion Size: 1 medium peach

Preparation: Enjoyed fresh, used in fruit salads, or blended into smoothies.

Earlitreat Peach

GI: 42

GL: 5 (per medium-sized peach)

Portion Size: 1 medium peach

Preparation: Eaten fresh, used in desserts, or added to yogurt.

Biscoe Peach

GI: 43

GL: 5 (per medium-sized peach)

Portion Size: 1 medium peach

Preparation: Enjoyed fresh, used in baking, or sliced for snacks.

Candor Peach

GI: 41

GL: 5 (per medium-sized peach)

Portion Size: 1 medium peach

Preparation: Eaten fresh, used in fruit salads, or blended into smoothies.

Diamond Princess Peach

GI: 40

GL: 5 (per medium-sized peach)

Portion Size: 1 medium peach

Preparation: Enjoyed fresh, used in desserts, or added to salads.

Early Star Peach

GI: 42

GL: 5 (per medium-sized peach)

Portion Size: 1 medium peach

Preparation: Eaten fresh, used in baking, or sliced for snacks.

Earlitreat Peach

GI: 43

GL: 5 (per medium-sized peach)

Portion Size: 1 medium peach

Preparation: Enjoyed fresh, used in fruit salads, or blended into smoothies.

Fireprince Peach

GI: 41

GL: 5 (per medium-sized peach)

Portion Size: 1 medium peach

Preparation: Eaten fresh, used in desserts, or added to yogurt.

Nuts

Almonds

GI: 0 (low GI)

GL: N/A

Portion Size: 1 ounce (about 23 almonds)

Preparation: Eaten raw, roasted, or used in baking and salads.

Walnuts

GI: 0 (low GI)

GL: N/A

Portion Size: 1 ounce (about 14 halves)

Preparation: Eaten raw, toasted, added to oatmeal, or used in baking.

Pistachios

GI: 0 (low GI)

GL: N/A

Portion Size: 1 ounce (about 49 kernels)

Preparation: Eaten raw, roasted, added to salads, or used in desserts.

Cashews

GI: 0 (low GI)

GL: N/A

Portion Size: 1 ounce (about 18 nuts)

Preparation: Eaten raw, roasted, used in stir-fries, or ground into nut butter.

Brazil Nuts

GI: 0 (low GI)

GL: N/A

Portion Size: 1 ounce (about 6 nuts)

Preparation: Eaten raw, added to granola, or used in baking.

Hazelnuts

GI: 0 (low GI)

GL: N/A

Portion Size: 1 ounce (about 21 nuts)

Preparation: Eaten raw, roasted, or used in desserts and sauces.

Macadamia Nuts

GI: 0 (low GI)

GL: N/A

Portion Size: 1 ounce (about 10-12 nuts)

Preparation: Eaten raw, roasted, or used in baking and salads.

Pecans

GI: 0 (low GI)

GL: N/A

Portion Size: 1 ounce (about 19 halves)

Preparation: Eaten raw, roasted, added to pies, or used in salads.

Pine Nuts

GI: 0 (low GI)

GL: N/A

Portion Size: 1 ounce (about 167 kernels)

Preparation: Eaten raw, toasted, used in pesto sauce, or sprinkled on salads.

Chestnuts

GI: 54

GL: 12 (per 100g serving)

Portion Size: 1 ounce (about 3 nuts)

Preparation: Roasted, boiled, or used in stuffing and soups.

Peanuts

GI: 14

GL: 1 (per 1 ounce)

Portion Size: 1 ounce (about 28 peanuts)

Preparation: Eaten raw, roasted, used in peanut butter, or added to stir-fries.

Coconut

GI: 45

GL: 3 (per 2 tablespoons shredded)

Portion Size: 2 tablespoons shredded

Preparation: Used in cooking, baking, or eaten raw.

Hickory Nuts

GI: 0 (low GI)

GL: N/A

Portion Size: 1 ounce (about 19 halves)

Preparation: Eaten raw or roasted, used in baking.

Black Walnuts

GI: 0 (low GI)

GL: N/A

Portion Size: 1 ounce (about 7 nuts)

Preparation: Eaten raw or roasted, used in baking.

Ginkgo Nuts

GI: 15

GL: 1 (per 100g serving)

Portion Size: 1 ounce (about 14 nuts)

Preparation: Cooked, added to dishes, or used in soups and desserts.

Acorns

GI: 0 (low GI)

GL: N/A

Portion Size: Varies

Preparation: Processed to remove bitter tannins, roasted, or ground into flour.

Butternuts

GI: 0 (low GI)

GL: N/A

Portion Size: 1 ounce (about 6 halves)

Preparation: Eaten raw or roasted, used in baking.

Beechnuts

GI: 0 (low GI)

GL: N/A

Portion Size: Varies

Preparation: Roasted, eaten raw, or used in cooking.

Butter Nuts

GI: 0 (low GI)

GL: N/A

Portion Size: 1 ounce (about 10 halves)

Preparation: Eaten raw or roasted, used in baking.

English Walnuts

GI: 0 (low GI)

GL: N/A

Portion Size: 1 ounce (about 14 halves)

Preparation: Eaten raw or roasted, used in baking and salads.

Heartnuts

GI: 0 (low GI)

GL: N/A

Portion Size: 1 ounce (about 8 halves)

Preparation: Eaten raw or roasted, used in baking.

Hicans

GI: 0 (low GI)

GL: N/A

Portion Size: 1 ounce (about 3 nuts)

Preparation: Eaten raw or roasted, used in baking.

Pinon Nuts

GI: 0 (low GI)

GL: N/A

Portion Size: 1 ounce (about 167 kernels)

Preparation: Eaten raw, toasted, used in cooking, or ground into flour.

Shagbark Hickory Nuts

GI: 0 (low GI)

GL: N/A

Portion Size: 1 ounce (about 19 halves)

Preparation: Eaten raw or roasted, used in baking.

American Beech Nuts

GI: 0 (low GI)

GL: N/A

Portion Size: Varies

Preparation: Roasted, eaten raw, or used in cooking.

American Hazelnuts

GI: 0 (low GI)

GL: N/A

Portion Size: 1 ounce (about 21 nuts)

Preparation: Eaten raw or roasted, used in baking.

Chinquapin Nuts

GI: 0 (low GI)

GL: N/A

Portion Size: Varies

Preparation: Eaten raw or roasted.

Japanese Walnut

GI: 0 (low GI)

GL: N/A

Portion Size: 1 ounce (about 10 halves)

Preparation: Eaten raw or roasted, used in baking.

Texas Black Walnut

GI: 0 (low GI)

GL: N/A

Portion Size: 1 ounce (about 7 nuts)

Preparation: Eaten raw or roasted, used in baking.

English Walnuts

GI: 0 (low GI)

GL: N/A

Portion Size: 1 ounce (about 14 halves)

Preparation: Eaten raw or roasted, used in baking and salads.

Legumes

Lentils (Green)

GI: 32

GL: 5 (per 150g cooked)

Portion Size: 1/2 cup cooked

Preparation: Boiled for salads, soups, or stews.

Chickpeas (Garbanzo Beans)

GI: 28

GL: 6 (per 150g cooked)

Portion Size: 1/2 cup cooked

Preparation: Cooked for hummus, curries, or roasted as snacks.

Black Beans

GI: 30

GL: 7 (per 150g cooked)

Portion Size: 1/2 cup cooked

Preparation: Used in soups, salads, or Mexican dishes like burritos.

Kidney Beans

GI: 29

GL: 7 (per 150g cooked)

Portion Size: 1/2 cup cooked

Preparation: Added to chili, salads, or mixed bean dishes.

Navy Beans

GI: 31

GL: 6 (per 150g cooked)

Portion Size: 1/2 cup cooked

Preparation: Used in baked beans, soups, or stews.

Pinto Beans

GI: 45

GL: 9 (per 150g cooked)

Portion Size: 1/2 cup cooked

Preparation: Used in Mexican cuisine, refried beans, or added to salads.

Mung Beans

GI: 25

GL: 4 (per 150g cooked)

Portion Size: 1/2 cup cooked

Preparation: Sprouted in salads, cooked in curries, or stir-fried.

Split Peas (Yellow)

GI: 25

GL: 4 (per 150g cooked)

Portion Size: 1/2 cup cooked

Preparation: Used in soups, stews, or mashed for spreads.

Cannellini Beans

GI: 31

GL: 7 (per 150g cooked)

Portion Size: 1/2 cup cooked

Preparation: Added to salads, soups, or pasta dishes.

Lima Beans

GI: 32

GL: 6 (per 150g cooked)

Portion Size: 1/2 cup cooked

Preparation: Used in succotash, stews, or casseroles.

Adzuki Beans

GI: 19

GL: 3 (per 150g cooked)

Portion Size: 1/2 cup cooked

Preparation: Sweetened for red bean paste, used in desserts, or added to salads.

Black-eyed Peas

GI: 33

GL: 6 (per 150g cooked)

Portion Size: 1/2 cup cooked

Preparation: Used in Southern dishes, salads, or stews.

Chana Dal

GI: 8

GL: 1 (per 150g cooked)

Portion Size: 1/2 cup cooked

Preparation: Used in Indian cuisine, soups, or curries.

French Lentils (Puy Lentils)

GI: 25

GL: 3 (per 150g cooked)

Portion Size: 1/2 cup cooked

Preparation: Used in salads, soups, or as a side dish.

Red Lentils

GI: 21

GL: 5 (per 150g cooked)

Portion Size: 1/2 cup cooked

Preparation: Used in curries, soups, or as a thickener.

Cowpeas (Black-eyed Cowpeas)

GI: 31

GL: 6 (per 150g cooked)

Portion Size: 1/2 cup cooked

Preparation: Used in Southern dishes, salads, or stews.

Great Northern Beans

GI: 31

GL: 6 (per 150g cooked)

Portion Size: 1/2 cup cooked

Preparation: Added to casseroles, soups, or salads.

Lentils (Brown)

GI: 33

GL: 5 (per 150g cooked)

Portion Size: 1/2 cup cooked

Preparation: Used in stews, soups, or mixed with rice.

Moth Beans

GI: 28

GL: 5 (per 150g cooked)

Portion Size: 1/2 cup cooked

Preparation: Used in curries, soups, or salads.

Peas (Green)

GI: 51

GL: 4 (per 150g cooked)

Portion Size: 1/2 cup cooked

Preparation: Used as a side dish, in salads, or added to stir-fries.

Soybeans

GI: 16

GL: 2 (per 150g cooked)

Portion Size: 1/2 cup cooked

Preparation: Used in tofu, edamame, or cooked in soups and stews.

Urad Dal (Black Gram)

GI: 30

GL: 6 (per 150g cooked)

Portion Size: 1/2 cup cooked

Preparation: Used in Indian cuisine, soups, or stews.

Anasazi Beans

GI: 29

GL: 6 (per 150g cooked)

Portion Size: 1/2 cup cooked

Preparation: Used in Southwestern cuisine, salads, or soups.

Fava Beans

GI: 33

GL: 7 (per 150g cooked)

Portion Size: 1/2 cup cooked

Preparation: Used in Mediterranean dishes, soups, or mashed as a spread.

Green Lentils

GI: 30

GL: 5 (per 150g cooked)

Portion Size: 1/2 cup cooked

Preparation: Used in salads, soups, or mixed with grains.

Lentils (Black)

GI: 30

GL: 5 (per 150g cooked)

Portion Size: 1/2 cup cooked

Preparation: Used in Indian cuisine, soups, or stews.

Lentils (Red)

GI: 21

GL: 5 (per 150g cooked)

Portion Size: 1/2 cup cooked

Preparation: Used in curries, soups, or mixed with rice.

Pink Beans

GI: 39

GL: 7 (per 150g cooked)

Portion Size: 1/2 cup cooked

Preparation: Used in Latin American cuisine, soups, or stews.

Pulses (Mixed Beans)

GI: 30

GL: 6 (per 150g cooked)

Portion Size: 1/2 cup cooked

Preparation: Used in mixed bean salads, soups, or stews.

Soybeans (Green)

GI: 18

GL: 3 (per 150g cooked)

Portion Size: 1/2 cup cooked

Preparation: Used in Asian cuisine, salads, or stir-fries.

Lentils

Green Lentils

GI: 30

GL: 5 (per 150g cooked)

Portion Size: 1/2 cup cooked

Preparation: Used in salads, soups, or mixed with grains.

Brown Lentils

GI: 33

GL: 5 (per 150g cooked)

Portion Size: 1/2 cup cooked

Preparation: Used in stews, soups, or mixed with rice.

Red Lentils

GI: 21

GL: 5 (per 150g cooked)

Portion Size: 1/2 cup cooked

Preparation: Used in curries, soups, or as a thickener.

French Lentils (Puy Lentils)

GI: 25

GL: 3 (per 150g cooked)

Portion Size: 1/2 cup cooked

Preparation: Used in salads, soups, or as a side dish.

Black Lentils

GI: 30

GL: 5 (per 150g cooked)

Portion Size: 1/2 cup cooked

Preparation: Used in Indian cuisine, soups, or stews.

Yellow Lentils (Toor Dal)

GI: 22

GL: 4 (per 150g cooked)

Portion Size: 1/2 cup cooked

Preparation: Used in Indian cuisine, soups, or curries.

Beluga Lentils

GI: 29

GL: 5 (per 150g cooked)

Portion Size: 1/2 cup cooked

Preparation: Used in salads, side dishes, or as a base for veggie burgers.

Masoor Dal (Red Split Lentils)

GI: 25

GL: 4 (per 150g cooked)

Portion Size: 1/2 cup cooked

Preparation: Used in Indian cuisine, soups, or curries.

Black-eyed Pea Lentils

GI: 29

GL: 5 (per 150g cooked)

Portion Size: 1/2 cup cooked

Preparation: Used in Southern cuisine, salads, or stews.

Petite Golden Lentils

GI: 21

GL: 3 (per 150g cooked)

Portion Size: 1/2 cup cooked

Preparation: Used in salads, soups, or mixed with rice dishes.

Coral Lentils

GI: 29

GL: 5 (per 150g cooked)

Portion Size: 1/2 cup cooked

Preparation: Used in salads, soups, or stews.

Green Pea Lentils

GI: 22

GL: 4 (per 150g cooked)

Portion Size: 1/2 cup cooked

Preparation: Used in salads, soups, or mixed with grains.

Spanish Pardina Lentils

GI: 29

GL: 5 (per 150g cooked)

Portion Size: 1/2 cup cooked

Preparation: Used in stews, soups, or as a side dish.

Caviar Lentils

GI: 29

GL: 5 (per 150g cooked)

Portion Size: 1/2 cup cooked

Preparation: Used in salads, side dishes, or as a base for vegetarian patties.

Petite Crimson Lentils

GI: 22

GL: 4 (per 150g cooked)

Portion Size: 1/2 cup cooked

Preparation: Used in salads, soups, or mixed with rice dishes.

French Green Lentils

GI: 25

GL: 3 (per 150g cooked)

Portion Size: 1/2 cup cooked

Preparation: Used in salads, soups, or as a side dish.

Madagascar Pink Lentils

GI: 29

GL: 5 (per 150g cooked)

Portion Size: 1/2 cup cooked

Preparation: Used in stews, soups, or as a side dish.

Black Beluga Lentils

GI: 30

GL: 5 (per 150g cooked)

Portion Size: 1/2 cup cooked

Preparation: Used in salads, side dishes, or as a base for veggie burgers.

Petite Golden Lentils

GI: 21

GL: 3 (per 150g cooked)

Portion Size: 1/2 cup cooked

Preparation: Used in salads, soups, or mixed with rice dishes.

Petite Crimson Lentils

GI: 22

GL: 4 (per 150g cooked)

Portion Size: 1/2 cup cooked

Preparation: Used in salads, soups, or mixed with rice dishes.

Petite Black Lentils

GI: 29

GL: 5 (per 150g cooked)

Portion Size: 1/2 cup cooked

Preparation: Used in salads, side dishes, or as a base for veggie burgers.

Petite Green Lentils

GI: 30

GL: 5 (per 150g cooked)

Portion Size: 1/2 cup cooked

Preparation: Used in salads, soups, or mixed with grains.

Red Chief Lentils

GI: 21

GL: 3 (per 150g cooked)

Portion Size: 1/2 cup cooked

Preparation: Used in curries, soups, or as a thickener.

Richlea Lentils

GI: 29

GL: 5 (per 150g cooked)

Portion Size: 1/2 cup cooked

Preparation: Used in stews, soups, or as a side dish.

Spanish Brown Lentils

GI: 33

GL: 5 (per 150g cooked)

Portion Size: 1/2 cup cooked

Preparation: Used in stews, soups, or mixed with rice dishes.

Petite Golden Lentils

GI: 21

GL: 3 (per 150g cooked)

Portion Size: 1/2 cup cooked

Preparation: Used in salads, soups, or mixed with rice dishes.

Petite Crimson Lentils

GI: 22

GL: 4 (per 150g cooked)

Portion Size: 1/2 cup cooked

Preparation: Used in salads, soups, or mixed with rice dishes.

Petite Black Lentils

GI: 29

GL: 5 (per 150g cooked)

Portion Size: 1/2 cup cooked

Preparation: Used in salads, side dishes, or as a base for veggie burgers.

Petite Green Lentils

GI: 30

GL: 5 (per 150g cooked)

Portion Size: 1/2 cup cooked

Preparation: Used in salads, soups, or mixed with grains.

Petite Yellow Lentils

GI: 22

GL: 4 (per 150g cooked)

Portion Size: 1/2 cup cooked

Preparation: Used in salads, soups, or mixed with rice dishes.

Varieties of Chickpeas

Kabuli Chickpeas (Garbanzo Beans)

GI: 28

GL: 6 (per 150g cooked)

Portion Size: 1/2 cup cooked

Preparation: Cooked for hummus, curries, or roasted for snacks.

Desi Chickpeas (Bengal Gram)

GI: 33

GL: 9 (per 150g cooked)

Portion Size: 1/2 cup cooked

Preparation: Used in Indian dishes like chana masala or soups.

Black Chickpeas (Kala Chana)

GI: 33

GL: 9 (per 150g cooked)

Portion Size: 1/2 cup cooked

Preparation: Used in Indian cuisine, salads, or curries.

Green Chickpeas

GI: 35

GL: 8 (per 150g cooked)

Portion Size: 1/2 cup cooked

Preparation: Used in salads, stir-fries, or as a snack.

Red Chickpeas

GI: 35

GL: 8 (per 150g cooked)

Portion Size: 1/2 cup cooked

Preparation: Used in salads, stews, or soups.

White Chickpeas

GI: 35

GL: 8 (per 150g cooked)

Portion Size: 1/2 cup cooked

Preparation: Used in salads, curries, or soups.

Cream Chickpeas

GI: 35

GL: 8 (per 150g cooked)

Portion Size: 1/2 cup cooked

Preparation: Used in salads, curries, or soups.

Peanut Chickpeas

GI: 30

GL: 7 (per 150g cooked)

Portion Size: 1/2 cup cooked

Preparation: Added to salads, used in stews, or roasted as snacks.

Thin-skinned Chickpeas

GI: 35

GL: 8 (per 150g cooked)

Portion Size: 1/2 cup cooked

Preparation: Used in salads, curries, or soups.

Egyptian Chickpeas

GI: 35

GL: 8 (per 150g cooked)

Portion Size: 1/2 cup cooked

Preparation: Used in salads, curries, or soups.

Ethiopian Chickpeas

GI: 35

GL: 8 (per 150g cooked)

Portion Size: 1/2 cup cooked

Preparation: Used in salads, curries, or soups.

Sundried Chickpeas

GI: 35

GL: 8 (per 150g cooked)

Portion Size: 1/2 cup cooked

Preparation: Used in salads, soups, or curries.

Small Chickpeas

GI: 35

GL: 8 (per 150g cooked)

Portion Size: 1/2 cup cooked

Preparation: Used in salads, curries, or soups.

Large Chickpeas

GI: 35

GL: 8 (per 150g cooked)

Portion Size: 1/2 cup cooked

Preparation: Used in salads, curries, or soups.

Round Chickpeas

GI: 35

GL: 8 (per 150g cooked)

Portion Size: 1/2 cup cooked

Preparation: Used in salads, curries, or soups.

Flat Chickpeas

GI: 35

GL: 8 (per 150g cooked)

Portion Size: 1/2 cup cooked

Preparation: Used in salads, curries, or soups.

Hard Chickpeas

GI: 35

GL: 8 (per 150g cooked)

Portion Size: 1/2 cup cooked

Preparation: Used in salads, curries, or soups.

Soft Chickpeas

GI: 35

GL: 8 (per 150g cooked)

Portion Size: 1/2 cup cooked

Preparation: Used in salads, curries, or soups.

Brown Chickpeas

GI: 35

GL: 8 (per 150g cooked)

Portion Size: 1/2 cup cooked

Preparation: Used in salads, curries, or soups.

Yellow Chickpeas

GI: 35

GL: 8 (per 150g cooked)

Portion Size: 1/2 cup cooked

Preparation: Used in salads, curries, or soups.

Pink Chickpeas

GI: 35

GL: 8 (per 150g cooked)

Portion Size: 1/2 cup cooked

Preparation: Used in salads, curries, or soups.

Blue Chickpeas

GI: 35

GL: 8 (per 150g cooked)

Portion Size: 1/2 cup cooked

Preparation: Used in salads, curries, or soups.

Purple Chickpeas

GI: 35

GL: 8 (per 150g cooked)

Portion Size: 1/2 cup cooked

Preparation: Used in salads, curries, or soups.

Gray Chickpeas

GI: 35

GL: 8 (per 150g cooked)

Portion Size: 1/2 cup cooked

Preparation: Used in salads, curries, or soups.

Orange Chickpeas

GI: 35

GL: 8 (per 150g cooked)

Portion Size: 1/2 cup cooked

Preparation: Used in salads, curries, or soups.

Crimson Chickpeas

GI: 35

GL: 8 (per 150g cooked)

Portion Size: 1/2 cup cooked

Preparation: Used in salads, curries, or soups.

Green Chickpeas

GI: 35

GL: 8 (per 150g cooked)

Portion Size: 1/2 cup cooked

Preparation: Used in salads, stir-fries, or as a snack.

Cream Chickpeas

GI: 35

GL: 8 (per 150g cooked)

Portion Size: 1/2 cup cooked

Preparation: Used in salads, curries, or soups.

White Chickpeas

GI: 35

GL: 8 (per 150g cooked)

Portion Size: 1/2 cup cooked

Preparation: Used in salads, curries, or soups.

Black Chickpeas

GI: 33

GL: 9 (per 150g cooked)

Portion Size: 1/2 cup cooked

Preparation: Used in salads, curries, or soups.

Kidney Beans

Red Kidney Beans

GI: 27

GL: 8 (per 150g cooked)

Portion Size: 1/2 cup cooked

Preparation: Used in chili, soups, or salads.

Light Red Kidney Beans

GI: 27

GL: 8 (per 150g cooked)

Portion Size: 1/2 cup cooked

Preparation: Used in stews, salads, or as a side dish.

Dark Red Kidney Beans

GI: 27

GL: 8 (per 150g cooked)

Portion Size: 1/2 cup cooked

Preparation: Used in chili, soups, or salads.

White Kidney Beans (Cannellini Beans)

GI: 31

GL: 8 (per 150g cooked)

Portion Size: 1/2 cup cooked

Preparation: Used in Italian dishes, soups, or salads.

Black Kidney Beans

GI: 27

GL: 8 (per 150g cooked)

Portion Size: 1/2 cup cooked

Preparation: Used in Mexican cuisine, soups, or salads.

Speckled Kidney Beans

GI: 27

GL: 8 (per 150g cooked)

Portion Size: 1/2 cup cooked

Preparation: Used in stews, salads, or as a side dish.

Striped Kidney Beans

GI: 27

GL: 8 (per 150g cooked)

Portion Size: 1/2 cup cooked

Preparation: Used in chili, soups, or salads.

Light Speckled Kidney Beans

GI: 27

GL: 8 (per 150g cooked)

Portion Size: 1/2 cup cooked

Preparation: Used in stews, salads, or as a side dish.

Dark Speckled Kidney Beans

GI: 27

GL: 8 (per 150g cooked)

Portion Size: 1/2 cup cooked

Preparation: Used in chili, soups, or salads.

Cream Kidney Beans

GI: 27

GL: 8 (per 150g cooked)

Portion Size: 1/2 cup cooked

Preparation: Used in stews, salads, or as a side dish.

Yellow Kidney Beans

GI: 27

GL: 8 (per 150g cooked)

Portion Size: 1/2 cup cooked

Preparation: Used in curries, soups, or salads.

Purple Kidney Beans

GI: 27

GL: 8 (per 150g cooked)

Portion Size: 1/2 cup cooked

Preparation: Used in stews, salads, or as a side dish.

Golden Kidney Beans

GI: 27

GL: 8 (per 150g cooked)

Portion Size: 1/2 cup cooked

Preparation: Used in salads, soups, or as a side dish.

Soy Products

Tofu (Firm)

GI: 15

GL: 1 (per 150g)

Portion Size: 1/2 cup cubes

Preparation: Used in stir-fries, grilled, or added to salads.

Tofu (Silken)

GI: 15

GL: 1 (per 150g)

Portion Size: 1/2 cup cubes

Preparation: Blended into smoothies, used in desserts, or as a base for sauces.

Edamame

GI: 15

GL: 1 (per 150g)

Portion Size: 1/2 cup cooked

Preparation: Boiled or steamed and served as a snack or added to salads.

Tempeh

GI: 35

GL: 4 (per 150g)

Portion Size: 1/2 cup cubes

Preparation: Marinated and grilled, added to stir-fries, or used in sandwiches.

Soy Milk (Unsweetened)

GI: 34

GL: 4 (per 1 cup)

Portion Size: 1 cup

Preparation: Consumed as a dairy milk alternative or used in cooking/baking.

Miso

GI: 25

GL: 2 (per tablespoon)

Portion Size: 1 tablespoon

Preparation: Used in soups, marinades, or as a seasoning paste.

Soy Sauce (Low Sodium)

GI: 36

GL: 0 (per tablespoon)

Portion Size: 1 tablespoon

Preparation: Used as a condiment or flavor enhancer in various dishes.

Soybean Sprouts

GI: 25

GL: 1 (per 150g)

Portion Size: 1/2 cup

Preparation: Added to salads, stir-fries, or used in wraps.

Soy Yogurt (Plain, Unsweetened)

GI: 33

GL: 4 (per 1 cup)

Portion Size: 1 cup

Preparation: Consumed as a dairy yogurt alternative or used in smoothies.

Soy Flour

GI: 35

GL: 4 (per 1/4 cup)

Portion Size: 1/4 cup

Preparation: Used in baking recipes or as a thickening agent in sauces.

Soy Protein Powder

GI: 25

GL: 1 (per scoop)

Portion Size: 1 scoop

Preparation: Added to smoothies or used as a protein supplement.

Soy Nuts

GI: 20

GL: 1 (per 1/4 cup)

Portion Size: 1/4 cup

Preparation: Roasted and consumed as a snack.

Soy Cheese

GI: 30

GL: 1 (per slice)

Portion Size: 1 slice

Preparation: Used as a topping on pizzas, sandwiches, or in casseroles.

Textured Vegetable Protein (TVP)

GI: 35

GL: 3 (per 1/4 cup)

Portion Size: 1/4 cup dry

Preparation: Rehydrated and used in vegetarian dishes or as a meat substitute.

Soy Ice Cream

GI: 50

GL: 6 (per 1/2 cup)

Portion Size: 1/2 cup

Preparation: Consumed as a dairy ice cream alternative.

Soy Butter

GI: 20

GL: 1 (per tablespoon)

Portion Size: 1 tablespoon

Preparation: Used as a spread or in baking/cooking.

Soybean Oil

GI: 0 (Source of fat, no GI)

GL: 0 (Source of fat, no GL)

Portion Size: Used for cooking/frying.

Soy-based Veggie Burgers

GI: 30

GL: 4 (per patty)

Portion Size: 1 patty

Preparation: Grilled or pan-fried and used as a meat alternative.

Soy-based Hot Dogs

GI: 18

GL: 2 (per hot dog)

Portion Size: 1 hot dog

Preparation: Grilled or cooked and used as a meat alternative.

Soy-based Deli Slices

GI: 15

GL: 1 (per serving)

Portion Size: 1 serving

Preparation: Used in sandwiches or wraps.

Soy Jerky

GI: 25

GL: 1 (per serving)

Portion Size: 1 serving

Preparation: Consumed as a snack.

Soy-based Bacon

GI: 25

GL: 2 (per serving)

Portion Size: 1 serving

Preparation: Pan-fried and used as a bacon substitute.

Soy-based Sausages

GI: 25

GL: 3 (per sausage)

Portion Size: 1 sausage

Preparation: Grilled or cooked and used as a sausage alternative.

Soy-based Chicken Strips

GI: 20

GL: 1 (per serving)

Portion Size: 1 serving

Preparation: Cooked and used in various recipes.

Soy-based Ground Meat

GI: 30

GL: 2 (per serving)

Portion Size: 1 serving

Preparation: Used in recipes that call for ground meat.

Soy-based Meatballs

GI: 25

GL: 2 (per serving)

Portion Size: 1 serving

Preparation: Used in pasta dishes or as appetizers.

Soy-based Chicken Nuggets

GI: 25

GL: 2 (per serving)

Portion Size: 1 serving

Preparation: Baked or fried and consumed as a snack or meal.

Soy-based Fish Fillets

GI: 20

GL: 1 (per serving)

Portion Size: 1 serving

Preparation: Cooked and used as a fish substitute.

Soy-based Seafood

GI: 18

GL: 1 (per serving)

Portion Size: 1 serving

Preparation: Used in dishes that traditionally call for seafood.

Soy-based Eggs (Vegan)

GI: 20

GL: 1 (per serving)

Portion Size: 1 serving

Preparation: Used in recipes that call for eggs.

Tofu Group

Tempeh

GI: Around 35

Portion: 100g

Preparation: Marinate tempeh in a mix of soy sauce, garlic, and ginger, then pan-fry until golden.

Edamame

GI: Around 30

Portion: 1 cup (cooked)

Preparation: Boil or steam edamame pods until tender, then sprinkle with sea salt.

Silken Tofu

GI: Around 15

Portion: 1/2 cup

Preparation: Blend silken tofu with fruits for a creamy smoothie base or use as a thickener in soups.

Firm Tofu

GI: Around 15

Portion: 100g

Preparation: Press and cube firm tofu, then stir-fry with vegetables and your choice of sauce.

Tofu Shirataki Noodles

GI: Around 20

Portion: 1 package

Preparation: Rinse noodles well, then stir-fry with vegetables and protein for a low-carb noodle dish.

Smoked Tofu

GI: Around 15

Portion: 100g

Preparation: Slice smoked tofu and pan-sear until crispy, then serve with salads or sandwiches.

Tofu Skin (Yuba)

GI: Around 20

Portion: 50g

Preparation: Use tofu skin as a wrapper for spring rolls or slice into strips for stir-fries.

Tofu Burgers/Patties

GI: Around 20

Portion: 1 patty

Preparation: Mix tofu with spices and breadcrumbs, then grill or bake for a healthy burger alternative.

Tofu Scramble

GI: Around 15

Portion: 100g

Preparation: Crumble tofu and sauté with vegetables and turmeric for a tasty breakfast scramble.

Tofu Frittata

GI: Around 15

Portion: 1 slice

Preparation: Combine tofu with veggies and bake for a delicious, protein-rich frittata.

Tofu Salad

GI: Around 15

Portion: 100g

Preparation: Cube tofu and mix with fresh greens, tomatoes, and a light vinaigrette.

Tofu Kebabs

GI: Around 20

Portion: 100g

Preparation: Skewer marinated tofu cubes with veggies and grill for flavorful kebabs.

Tofu Stir-fry

GI: Around 15

Portion: 100g

Preparation: Stir-fry tofu with broccoli, bell peppers, and a savory sauce for a quick meal.

Tofu Soup

GI: Around 15

Portion: 1 bowl

Preparation: Simmer tofu cubes in a vegetable broth with mushrooms and greens for a comforting soup.

Tofu Tacos

GI: Around 20

Portion: 2 tacos

Preparation: Crumble tofu and cook with taco seasoning, then fill taco shells with tofu mixture and favorite toppings.

Tofu Curry

GI: Around 15

Portion: 100g

Preparation: Simmer tofu in a flavorful curry sauce with coconut milk and vegetables.

Tofu Skewers

GI: Around 20

Portion: 2 skewers

Preparation: Thread tofu cubes onto skewers with pineapple and bell peppers, then grill for a sweet and savory dish.

Tofu Sushi Rolls

GI: Around 20

Portion: 6 pieces

Preparation: Use tofu strips along with vegetables to roll sushi, served with soy sauce and wasabi.

Tofu Smoothie Bowl

GI: Around 15

Portion: 1 bowl

Preparation: Blend silken tofu with fruits and top with granola and nuts for a nutritious breakfast bowl.

Tofu Satay

GI: Around 20

Portion: 100g

Preparation: Marinate tofu in a peanut-based sauce, then grill or bake for tasty satay skewers.

Tofu Stuffed Peppers

GI: Around 20

Portion: 1 pepper

Preparation: Stuff halved bell peppers with tofu, vegetables, and cheese, then bake until tender.

Tofu Quiche

GI: Around 15

Portion: 1 slice

Preparation: Mix tofu with veggies and bake in a pie crust for a satisfying quiche.

Tofu and Veggie Skillet

GI: Around 15

Portion: 100g

Preparation: Sauté tofu with assorted veggies in a skillet and season with herbs and spices.

Tofu Pad Thai

GI: Around 20

Portion: 1 serving

Preparation: Stir-fry tofu, rice noodles, and veggies with a tangy Pad Thai sauce.

Tofu Spring Rolls

GI: Around 20

Portion: 2 rolls

Preparation: Wrap tofu strips, veggies, and herbs in rice paper sheets for fresh spring rolls.

Tofu and Lentil Soup

GI: Around 15

Portion: 1 bowl

Preparation: Combine tofu cubes with lentils, vegetables, and broth for a hearty soup.

Tofu Skillet Hash

GI: Around 15

Portion: 100g

Preparation: Cube tofu and sauté with potatoes and onions for a flavorful breakfast hash.

Tofu Pasta Sauce

GI: Around 15

Portion: 1 cup

Preparation: Blend tofu with tomatoes and herbs for a creamy pasta sauce.

Tofu Lettuce Wraps

GI: Around 20

Portion: 2 wraps

Preparation: Fill lettuce leaves with tofu, water chestnuts, and a flavorful sauce for a light meal.

Tofu Stew

GI: Around 15

Portion: 1 bowl

Preparation: Simmer tofu with root vegetables and herbs for a comforting stew.

Dairy Products

Plain Greek Yogurt

GI: Around 11

GL: 4 (per 6 ounces)

Portion: 6 ounces

Preparation: Enjoy as is or use as a base for smoothies or dressings.

Cottage Cheese

GI: Around 10

GL: 3 (per 1/2 cup)

Portion: 1/2 cup

Preparation: Have it plain or mix with fruits or vegetables for a savory option.

Unsweetened Almond Milk

GI: Around 25

GL: 1 (per cup)

Portion: 1 cup

Preparation: Use in smoothies, cereal, or as a dairy-free alternative in recipes.

Plain Kefir

GI: Around 20

GL: 8 (per cup)

Portion: 1 cup

Preparation: Consume as a beverage or blend into smoothies.

Plain Skyr

GI: Around 30

GL: 4 (per 6 ounces)

Portion: 6 ounces

Preparation: Enjoy plain or mix with fruits for added flavor.

Sour Cream (Full Fat)

GI: Around 20

GL: 1 (per tablespoon)

Portion: 1 tablespoon

Preparation: Use as a topping for savory dishes or in dips.

Plain Whole Milk

GI: Around 27

GL: 5 (per cup)

Portion: 1 cup

Preparation: Drink as is or use in cooking and baking.

Buttermilk

GI: Around 15

GL: 3 (per cup)

Portion: 1 cup

Preparation: Use in baking or marinating meats.

Unsweetened Soy Milk

GI: Around 25

GL: 4 (per cup)

Portion: 1 cup

Preparation: Use in coffee, cereal, or as a dairy alternative in recipes.

Plain Ricotta Cheese

GI: Around 35

GL: 3 (per 1/2 cup)

Portion: 1/2 cup

Preparation: Use in savory or sweet dishes, or as a topping.

Plain Regular Yogurt

GI: Around 23

GL: 12 (per cup)

Portion: 1 cup

Preparation: Enjoy plain or use in marinades or dips.

Unsweetened Cashew Milk

GI: Around 25

GL: 1 (per cup)

Portion: 1 cup

Preparation: Use in cooking, baking, or as a non-dairy milk alternative.

Full-Fat Cream Cheese

GI: Around 15

GL: 1 (per tablespoon)

Portion: 1 tablespoon

Preparation: Use in spreads or as a topping for bagels.

Plain Hemp Milk

GI: Around 30

GL: 2 (per cup)

Portion: 1 cup

Preparation: Use in smoothies, cereal, or as a dairy substitute in recipes.

Plain Goat Cheese

GI: Around 30

GL: 1 (per ounce)

Portion: 1 ounce

Preparation: Use in salads, sandwiches, or as a topping.

Unsweetened Coconut Milk

GI: Around 20

GL: 1 (per cup)

Portion: 1 cup

Preparation: Use in cooking, baking, or as a dairy-free milk alternative.

Plain Buffalo Milk Yogurt

GI: Around 45

GL: 9 (per cup)

Portion: 1 cup

Preparation: Enjoy plain or mix with fruits for added flavor.

Plain Sheep Milk Yogurt

GI: Around 20

GL: 5 (per 6 ounces)

Portion: 6 ounces

Preparation: Enjoy plain or with added fruits.

Whole Milk Ricotta Cheese

GI: Around 45

GL: 5 (per 1/2 cup)

Portion: 1/2 cup

Preparation: Use in baking, as a topping, or in savory dishes.

Plain Labneh (strained yogurt)

GI: Around 30

GL: 6 (per 2 tablespoons)

Portion: 2 tablespoons

Preparation: Use as a spread or dip with added herbs or spices.

Full-Fat Plain Cream

GI: Around 20

GL: 1 (per tablespoon)

Portion: 1 tablespoon

Preparation: Use in cooking, baking, or as a topping.

Whole Milk Kefir

GI: Around 30

GL: 9 (per cup)

Portion: 1 cup

Preparation: Enjoy as a beverage or use in smoothies.

Plain Whole Milk Lassi

GI: Around 25

GL: 8 (per cup)

Portion: 1 cup

Preparation: Enjoy as a beverage or with added spices.

Quark Cheese

GI: Around 40

GL: 3 (per 1/2 cup)

Portion: 1/2 cup

Preparation: Use in recipes or enjoy plain with added fruits.

Full-Fat Plain Fromage Blanc

GI: Around 50

GL: 4 (per 2 tablespoons)

Portion: 2 tablespoons

Preparation: Use in recipes or enjoy as a topping.

Plain Full-Fat Greek Yogurt

GI: Around 11

GL: 4 (per 6 ounces)

Portion: 6 ounces

Preparation: Enjoy as is or use as a base for dips or dressings.

Whole Milk Cottage Cheese

GI: Around 10

GL: 3 (per 1/2 cup)

Portion: 1/2 cup

Preparation: Have it plain or mix with fruits for a snack.

Unsweetened Plain Yakult

GI: Around 30

GL: 5 (per bottle)

Portion: 1 bottle

Preparation: Drink as is for its probiotic benefits.

Full-Fat Plain Laban

GI: Around 25

GL: 6 (per cup)

Portion: 1 cup

Preparation: Enjoy as a beverage or use in savory dishes.

Plain Buffalo Milk Mozzarella Cheese

GI: Around 30

GL: 1 (per ounce)

Portion: 1 ounce

Preparation: Use in salads, pizzas, or as a topping.

Unsweetened Greek Yogurt

Regular Plain Yogurt

GI: Around 33

GL: 6 (per 6 ounces)

Portion: 6 ounces

Preparation: Enjoy as is or use in smoothies or dressings.

Cottage Cheese

GI: Around 10

GL: 3 (per 1/2 cup)

Portion: 1/2 cup

Preparation: Consume plain or mix with fruits for a satisfying snack.

Unsweetened Almond Milk

GI: Around 25

GL: 1 (per cup)

Portion: 1 cup

Preparation: Use in smoothies, cereal, or as a milk substitute in recipes.

Plain Kefir

GI: Around 20

GL: 8 (per cup)

Portion: 1 cup

Preparation: Enjoy as a beverage or blend into smoothies.

Plain Skyr

GI: Around 30

GL: 4 (per 6 ounces)

Portion: 6 ounces

Preparation: Enjoy plain or mix with fruits for added flavor.

Sour Cream (Full Fat)

GI: Around 20

GL: 1 (per tablespoon)

Portion: 1 tablespoon

Preparation: Use as a topping for savory dishes or in dips.

Whole Milk

GI: Around 27

GL: 5 (per cup)

Portion: 1 cup

Preparation: Drink as is or use in cooking and baking.

Buttermilk

GI: Around 15

GL: 3 (per cup)

Portion: 1 cup

Preparation: Use in baking or as a marinade for meats.

Unsweetened Soy Milk

GI: Around 25

GL: 4 (per cup)

Portion: 1 cup

Preparation: Use in coffee, cereal, or as a dairy alternative in recipes.

Plain Ricotta Cheese

GI: Around 35

GL: 3 (per 1/2 cup)

Portion: 1/2 cup

Preparation: Use in sweet or savory dishes, or as a topping.

Plain Regular Yogurt

GI: Around 23

GL: 12 (per cup)

Portion: 1 cup

Preparation: Enjoy plain or use in marinades or dips.

Unsweetened Cashew Milk

GI: Around 25

GL: 1 (per cup)

Portion: 1 cup

Preparation: Use in cooking, baking, or as a non-dairy milk alternative.

Full-Fat Cream Cheese

GI: Around 15

GL: 1 (per tablespoon)

Portion: 1 tablespoon

Preparation: Use in spreads or as a topping for bagels.

Plain Hemp Milk

GI: Around 30

GL: 2 (per cup)

Portion: 1 cup

Preparation: Use in smoothies, cereal, or as a dairy substitute in recipes.

Plain Goat Cheese

GI: Around 30

GL: 1 (per ounce)

Portion: 1 ounce

Preparation: Use in salads, sandwiches, or as a topping.

Unsweetened Coconut Milk

GI: Around 20

GL: 1 (per cup)

Portion: 1 cup

Preparation: Use in cooking, baking, or as a dairy-free milk alternative.

Plain Buffalo Milk Yogurt

GI: Around 45

GL: 9 (per cup)

Portion: 1 cup

Preparation: Enjoy plain or mix with fruits for added flavor.

Plain Sheep Milk Yogurt

GI: Around 20

GL: 5 (per 6 ounces)

Portion: 6 ounces

Preparation: Enjoy plain or with added fruits.

Whole Milk Ricotta Cheese

GI: Around 45

GL: 5 (per 1/2 cup)

Portion: 1/2 cup

Preparation: Use in baking, as a topping, or in savory dishes.

Plain Labneh (strained yogurt)

GI: Around 30

GL: 6 (per 2 tablespoons)

Portion: 2 tablespoons

Preparation: Use as a spread or dip with added herbs or spices.

Full-Fat Plain Cream

GI: Around 20

GL: 1 (per tablespoon)

Portion: 1 tablespoon

Preparation: Use in cooking, baking, or as a topping.

Whole Milk Kefir

GI: Around 30

GL: 9 (per cup)

Portion: 1 cup

Preparation: Enjoy as a beverage or use in smoothies.

Plain Whole Milk Lassi

GI: Around 25

GL: 8 (per cup)

Portion: 1 cup

Preparation: Enjoy as a beverage or with added spices.

Quark Cheese

GI: Around 40

GL: 3 (per 1/2 cup)

Portion: 1/2 cup

Preparation: Use in recipes or enjoy plain with added fruits.

Full-Fat Plain Fromage Blanc

GI: Around 50

GL: 4 (per 2 tablespoons)

Portion: 2 tablespoons

Preparation: Use in recipes or enjoy as a topping.

Plain Full-Fat Greek Yogurt

GI: Around 11

GL: 4 (per 6 ounces)

Portion: 6 ounces

Preparation: Enjoy as is or use as a base for dips or dressings.

Whole Milk Cottage Cheese

GI: Around 10

GL: 3 (per 1/2 cup)

Portion: 1/2 cup

Preparation: Have it plain or mix with fruits for a snack.

Unsweetened Plain Yakult

GI: Around 30

GL: 5 (per bottle)

Portion: 1 bottle

Preparation: Drink as is for its probiotic benefits.

Full-Fat Plain Laban

GI: Around 25

GL: 6 (per cup)

Portion: 1 cup

Preparation: Enjoy as a beverage or use in savory dishes.

Plain Buffalo Milk Mozzarella Cheese

GI: Around 30

GL: 1 (per ounce)

Portion: 1 ounce

Preparation: Use in salads, pizzas, or as a topping.

Bakery Products and Bread

White Bread

GL: 10

GI: 75

Portion Size: 1 slice (30 grams)

Preparation: No preparation required; serve as is or use for sandwiches.

Whole Wheat Bread

GL: 9

GI: 74

Portion Size: 1 slice (30 grams)

Preparation: Serve as is or toast for added crispness.

Multigrain Bread

GL: 9

GI: 75

Portion Size: 1 slice (30 grams)

Preparation: Use as a base for sandwiches or toast lightly.

Sourdough Bread

GL: 12

GI: 53

Portion Size: 1 slice (30 grams)

Preparation: Toast or serve alongside soups and salads.

Rye Bread

GL: 8

GI: 50

Portion Size: 1 slice (30 grams)

Preparation: Serve as is or lightly toast for added flavor.

Pumpernickel Bread

GL: 41

GI: 41

Portion Size: 1 slice (30 grams)

Preparation: Serve as is or use as a base for open-faced sandwiches.

French Baguette

GL: 20

GI: 95

Portion Size: 1 small piece (30 grams)

Preparation: Serve as is or toast for added crunchiness.

Ciabatta Bread

GL: 13

GI: 87

Portion Size: 1 slice (30 grams)

Preparation: Toast lightly or use for making paninis.

English Muffin

GL: 12

GI: 77

Portion Size: 1 muffin (60 grams)

Preparation: Toast and serve with butter or jam.

Croissant

GL: 17

GI: 67

Portion Size: 1 small croissant (40 grams)

Preparation: Warm in the oven for a flaky, buttery treat.

Brioche

GL: 13

GI: 64

Portion Size: 1 slice (30 grams)

Preparation: Enjoy as is or lightly toast for added richness.

Cinnamon Roll

GL: 28

GI: 77

Portion Size: 1 small roll (60 grams)

Preparation: Warm in the oven and enjoy as a sweet treat.

Bagel (Plain)

GL: 25

GI: 72

Portion Size: 1 small bagel (70 grams)

Preparation: Toast lightly and serve with cream cheese or toppings.

Flatbread

GL: 28

GI: 72

Portion Size: 1 piece (30 grams)

Preparation: Warm in a skillet or oven and use for wraps or as a side.

Naan Bread

GL: 38

GI: 72

Portion Size: 1 piece (30 grams)

Preparation: Warm in the oven and serve with curries or dips.

Tortilla (Flour)

GL: 30

GI: 30

Portion Size: 1 tortilla (30 grams)

Preparation: Heat on a skillet for a few seconds on each side and use for wraps or tacos.

Pita Bread

GL: 23

GI: 57

Portion Size: 1 round (30 grams)

Preparation: Warm in the oven or toaster and use for sandwiches or as a dipper.

Focaccia

GL: 14

GI: 68

Portion Size: 1 slice (30 grams)

Preparation: Enjoy as is or toast lightly with olive oil and herbs.

Panettone

GL: 70

GI: 70

Portion Size: 1 slice (30 grams)

Preparation: Serve as is or enjoy with coffee or tea during the holidays.

Zwieback

GL: 48

GI: 48

Portion Size: 1 slice (30 grams)

Preparation: Enjoy as a crispy snack or with toppings like jam or butter.

Matzo

GL: 12

GI: 12

Portion Size: 1 piece (30 grams)

Preparation: Serve as a traditional unleavened bread or use in recipes during Passover.

Muffin (Blueberry)

GL: 25

GI: 59

Portion Size: 1 small muffin (60 grams)

Preparation: Enjoy as is for a quick breakfast or snack.

Donut (Plain)

GL: 22

GI: 76

Portion Size: 1 small donut (40 grams)

Preparation: Enjoy as a sweet indulgence.

Scone (Plain)

GL: 25

GI: 92

Portion Size: 1 small scone (60 grams)

Preparation: Enjoy as is or with a spread of butter or jam.

Danish Pastry

GL: 24

GI: 59

Portion Size: 1 small pastry (60 grams)

Preparation: Serve as is for a sweet pastry treat.

Baguette (Whole Wheat)

GL: 12

GI: 65

Portion Size: 1 small piece (30 grams)

Preparation: Serve as is or lightly toast for added crunch.

Fruit Bread

GL: 14

GI: 64

Portion Size: 1 slice (30 grams)

Preparation: Serve as is or toast lightly for breakfast.

Pretzel (Soft)

GL: 12

GI: 83

Portion Size: 1 small pretzel (40 grams)

Preparation: Warm in the oven and enjoy as a savory snack.

Coffee Cake

GL: 26

GI: 70

Portion Size: 1 slice (30 grams)

Preparation: Serve as is or warm slightly before serving.

Cornbread

GL: 11

GI: 95

Portion Size: 1 piece (30 grams)

Preparation: Serve as is or with a drizzle of honey for added sweetness.

Biscuit

GL: 20

GI: 67

Portion Size: 1 small biscuit (30 grams)

Preparation: Serve as a side with butter or gravy.

English Scone

GL: 16

GI: 92

Portion Size: 1 small scone (60 grams)

Preparation: Enjoy as is or with clotted cream and jam.

Poppy Seed Muffin

GL: 27

GI: 58

Portion Size: 1 small muffin (60 grams)

Preparation: Enjoy as a quick snack or breakfast option.

Crumpet

GL: 15

GI: 69

Portion Size: 1 crumpet (30 grams)

Preparation: Toast lightly and serve with butter or jam.

Raisin Bread

GL: 11

GI: 64

Portion Size: 1 slice (30 grams)

Preparation: Serve as is or lightly toast for breakfast or snacks.

UNDERSTANDING HIGH-GLYCEMIC FOODS

High-glycemic foods are those that prompt a rapid spike in blood sugar levels after consumption due to their quick digestion and absorption. These foods rank high on the glycemic index (GI), a scale measuring the impact of carbohydrates on blood glucose levels. They're characterized by their ability to swiftly elevate blood sugar, causing a sudden surge followed by a rapid decline, potentially leading to fluctuations in energy levels and hunger.

Identifying High-Glycemic Foods to Limit or Avoid

White Bread and White Rice: Refined grains lacking fiber, which accelerates their breakdown and absorption, resulting in a rapid surge in blood sugar.

Processed Breakfast Cereals: Often loaded with sugars and lacking fiber, these cereals digest quickly, causing a rapid rise in blood glucose levels.

Sweetened Beverages: Sodas, energy drinks, and fruit juices with added sugars rapidly elevate blood sugar due to their high sugar content.

Candies and Sweets: Sweets with refined sugars, lacking fiber or protein, lead to a quick surge in blood glucose followed by a rapid drop.

Potatoes: While a staple, especially in their processed forms like mashed or instant potatoes, they have a high GI, affecting blood sugar levels significantly.

Instant Noodles and Pasta: Highly processed and lacking fiber, these carbohydrates rapidly break down into sugars, affecting blood sugar levels.

Snack Foods: Many packaged snacks like crackers, chips, and pretzels contain refined flours, leading to quick spikes in blood sugar.

Effects of High-Glycemic Foods on Blood Sugar Levels:

Consuming high-glycemic foods results in a rapid increase in blood sugar levels, causing the pancreas to release more insulin to regulate the surge. This sudden insulin release may lead to a subsequent drop in blood sugar, causing fatigue, hunger, and cravings for more high-glycemic foods. Over time, frequent consumption of these foods may contribute to insulin resistance, weight gain, and an increased risk of type 2 diabetes.

It's crucial to be mindful of high-glycemic foods, especially for individuals managing blood sugar levels or aiming for sustained energy throughout the day. Choosing low to moderate glycemic options, incorporating fiber-rich foods, lean proteins, and healthy fats into meals helps in stabilizing blood sugar levels and maintaining overall health.

Balancing high-glycemic foods with low-GI options, focusing on whole grains, vegetables, fruits, and lean proteins, contributes to better blood sugar control and sustained energy levels throughout the day. Awareness and moderation in consuming high-GI foods play a vital role in promoting overall health and well-being.

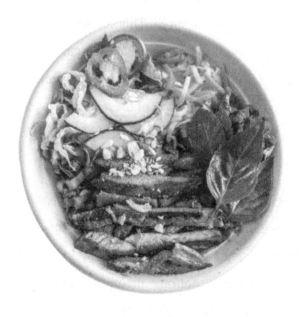

FLAVORFUL AND DELICIOUS RECIPES

Breakfast Recipes

Recipe 1: *Veggie Omelette with Whole Grain Toast*

Ingredients:

- 2 large eggs
- 1/4 cup diced bell peppers (red, green, yellow)
- 1/4 cup diced onions
- 1/4 cup chopped spinach
- 1 small tomato, diced
- 1 teaspoon olive oil
- Salt and pepper to taste
- 2 slices whole grain bread

Method:

1. In a bowl, whisk the eggs and season with salt and pepper.
2. Heat olive oil in a non-stick skillet over medium heat.
3. Add diced onions and bell peppers to the skillet. Sauté until they begin to soften.

4. Add chopped spinach and diced tomatoes to the skillet. Cook for another minute.

5. Pour the whisked eggs over the vegetables in the skillet.

6. Gently lift the edges of the omelette as it cooks to let uncooked eggs flow underneath.

7. Once the omelette is set, fold it in half and cook for another minute.

8. Toast two slices of whole grain bread.

Portion Size: 1 veggie omelette with 2 slices of whole grain toast

Nutrition Details: Approximately 300-350 calories per serving, depending on the size of the vegetables used. Provides a balanced mix of protein, healthy fats, fiber, vitamins, and minerals.

Recipe 2: *Greek Yogurt Parfait with Berries and Nuts*

Ingredients:

- 1 cup Greek yogurt (unsweetened)
- 1/2 cup mixed berries (strawberries, blueberries, raspberries)
- 1 tablespoon chopped almonds or walnuts
- 1 teaspoon honey or stevia (optional for sweetness)

Method:

1. In a glass or bowl, layer half of the Greek yogurt.
2. Add a layer of mixed berries on top of the yogurt.
3. Sprinkle a portion of chopped nuts over the berries.
4. Repeat the layering process with the remaining yogurt, berries, and nuts.
5. Drizzle honey or sprinkle stevia for added sweetness if desired.

Portion Size: 1 serving of Greek yogurt parfait

Nutrition Details: Approximately 250-300 calories per serving, rich in protein, healthy fats, antioxidants, and fiber. The berries offer natural sweetness and a low glycemic index, contributing to better blood sugar control.

Lunch Recipes

Recipe 3: *Grilled Chicken Salad with Quinoa*

Ingredients:

- 4 oz (113g) grilled chicken breast, sliced
- 2 cups mixed salad greens (spinach, kale, arugula)
- 1/2 cup cooked quinoa
- 1/4 cup sliced cucumbers
- 1/4 cup cherry tomatoes, halved
- 1/4 cup bell peppers (assorted colors), sliced
- 1 tablespoon olive oil
- 1 tablespoon balsamic vinegar
- Salt and pepper to taste

Method:

1. Season the grilled chicken breast with a pinch of salt and pepper.
2. Grill the chicken until fully cooked and slice it into strips.
3. In a mixing bowl, combine the mixed salad greens, cooked quinoa, sliced cucumbers, cherry tomatoes, and bell peppers.

4. Drizzle olive oil and balsamic vinegar over the salad mixture. Toss gently to coat the ingredients.

5. Place the sliced grilled chicken on top of the salad.

Portion Size: 1 serving of grilled chicken salad

Nutrition Details: Approximately 350-400 calories per serving, rich in lean protein, fiber, vitamins, and minerals. The quinoa provides complex carbohydrates and the salad offers a mix of nutrients for sustained energy.

Recipe 4: *Baked Salmon with Roasted Vegetables*

Ingredients:

- 4 oz (113g) salmon fillet
- 1 cup mixed vegetables (zucchini, bell peppers, onions)
- 1 tablespoon olive oil
- 1 teaspoon dried herbs (rosemary, thyme, or your choice)
- Salt and pepper to taste
- Lemon wedges for serving (optional)

Method:

1. Preheat the oven to 400°F (200°C).

2. Place the mixed vegetables on a baking sheet, drizzle with olive oil, and sprinkle with dried herbs, salt, and pepper. Toss to coat evenly.

3. Bake the vegetables for 15-20 minutes until they are tender and slightly golden.

4. Season the salmon fillet with salt and pepper.

5. Place the salmon on another baking sheet lined with parchment paper and bake for 12-15 minutes until cooked through.

6. Serve the baked salmon with the roasted vegetables and garnish with lemon wedges if desired.

Portion Size: 1 serving of baked salmon with roasted vegetables

Nutrition Details: Approximately 350-400 calories per serving. Rich in omega-3 fatty acids, protein, fiber, and essential nutrients. The combination of salmon and vegetables offers a nutrient-dense and low-glycemic meal beneficial for blood sugar control.

Dinner Recipes

Recipe 5: *Grilled Lemon Herb Chicken with Roasted Vegetables*

Ingredients:

- 4 oz (113g) chicken breast
- 1 tablespoon olive oil
- 1 teaspoon lemon zest
- 1 tablespoon lemon juice
- 1 teaspoon dried herbs (rosemary, thyme, or your choice)
- Salt and pepper to taste
- 1 cup mixed vegetables (bell peppers, zucchini, onions)
- Cooking spray

Method:

1. Preheat the grill to medium-high heat.
2. In a bowl, mix olive oil, lemon zest, lemon juice, dried herbs, salt, and pepper.
3. Coat the chicken breast with the mixture.

4. Grill the chicken for about 6-8 minutes per side or until fully cooked.

5. Meanwhile, preheat the oven to 400°F (200°C).

6. Toss the mixed vegetables with a bit of olive oil, salt, and pepper.

7. Spread the vegetables on a baking sheet lined with parchment paper and roast for 15-20 minutes until tender.

Portion Size: 1 serving of grilled lemon herb chicken with roasted vegetables

Nutrition Details: Approximately 300-350 calories per serving. Rich in lean protein, fiber, vitamins, and minerals. The combination of grilled chicken and roasted vegetables offers a balanced, low-glycemic meal.

Recipe 6: *Baked Herb-Crusted Salmon with Steamed Broccoli and Quinoa*

Ingredients:

- 4 oz (113g) salmon fillet
- 1 tablespoon olive oil
- 1 teaspoon dried herbs (parsley, dill, or your choice)
- Salt and pepper to taste
- 1 cup broccoli florets
- 1/2 cup cooked quinoa
- Lemon wedges for serving (optional)

Method:

- Preheat the oven to 400°F (200°C).
- Rub the salmon fillet with olive oil and sprinkle with dried herbs, salt, and pepper.
- Place the salmon on a baking sheet lined with parchment paper and bake for 12-15 minutes until cooked through.
- While the salmon is baking, steam the broccoli until tender.
- Cook the quinoa according to package instructions.

Portion Size: 1 serving of baked herb-crusted salmon with steamed broccoli and quinoa

Nutrition Details: Approximately 350-400 calories per serving. Rich in omega-3 fatty acids, protein, fiber, and essential nutrients. This meal offers a mix of protein, healthy fats, and complex carbohydrates, aiding in blood sugar regulation.

Snack Recipes

Recipe 7: *Greek Yogurt with Berries and Almonds*

Ingredients:

- 1/2 cup Greek yogurt (unsweetened)
- 1/4 cup mixed berries (strawberries, blueberries, raspberries)
- 1 tablespoon chopped almonds
- Method:
- In a bowl, place the Greek yogurt.
- Top it with mixed berries and chopped almonds.

Portion Size: 1 serving of Greek yogurt with berries and almonds

Nutrition Details: Approximately 150-200 calories per serving. Rich in protein, healthy fats, antioxidants, and fiber. The combination of Greek yogurt, berries, and almonds offers a mix of nutrients beneficial for blood sugar control.

Recipe 8: *Veggie Sticks with Hummus*

Ingredients:

- 1 medium carrot, cut into sticks
- 1 medium cucumber, cut into sticks
- 1/4 cup hummus (homemade or store-bought)

Method:

1. Cut the carrot and cucumber into sticks.
2. Serve the veggie sticks with hummus for dipping.

Portion Size: 1 serving of veggie sticks with hummus

Nutrition Details: Approximately 100-150 calories per serving. Rich in fiber, vitamins, minerals, and healthy fats. The combination of vegetables and hummus provides a satisfying snack with low glycemic impact.

Dessert Recipes

Recipe 9: *Baked Apples with Cinnamon and Walnuts*

Ingredients:

- 2 medium-sized apples (such as Granny Smith or Honeycrisp)
- 2 tablespoons chopped walnuts
- 1 teaspoon cinnamon
- 1 teaspoon unsalted butter (optional)

Method:

1. Preheat the oven to 375°F (190°C).
2. Core the apples, removing the seeds and creating a hollow space in the center.
3. Mix chopped walnuts with cinnamon.
4. Stuff each apple with the walnut-cinnamon mixture.
5. Optionally, top each apple with a small knob of unsalted butter.
6. Place the stuffed apples on a baking sheet lined with parchment paper and bake for 25-30 minutes until tender.

Portion Size: 1 baked apple

Nutrition Details: Approximately 150-200 calories per serving. Rich in fiber, antioxidants, and healthy fats from walnuts. This dessert provides natural sweetness from apples without added sugars.

Recipe 10: Greek Yogurt Berry Parfait

Ingredients:

- 1 cup Greek yogurt (unsweetened)
- 1/2 cup mixed berries (strawberries, blueberries, raspberries)
- 1 tablespoon crushed nuts (almonds, walnuts, or your choice)
- 1 teaspoon honey or stevia (optional for sweetness)

Method:

1. In a glass or bowl, layer half of the Greek yogurt.
2. Add a layer of mixed berries on top of the yogurt.
3. Sprinkle a portion of crushed nuts over the berries.
4. Repeat the layering process with the remaining yogurt, berries, and nuts.
5. Drizzle honey or sprinkle stevia for added sweetness if desired.

Portion Size: 1 serving of Greek yogurt berry parfait

Nutrition Details: Approximately 200-250 calories per serving. Rich in protein, antioxidants, fiber, and essential nutrients. This dessert offers natural sweetness from berries and a protein boost from Greek yogurt.

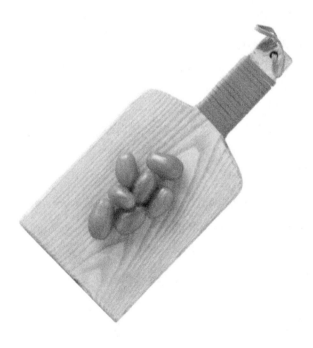

7-Day Meal Plan

Breakfast: Veggie Omelette with Whole Grain Toast

Lunch: Grilled Chicken Salad with Quinoa

Dinner: Grilled Lemon Herb Chicken with Roasted Vegetables

Snack: Greek Yogurt with Berries and Almonds

Dessert: Baked Apples with Cinnamon and Walnuts

Breakfast: Greek Yogurt Parfait with Berries and Nuts

Lunch: Baked Salmon with Roasted Vegetables

Dinner: Baked Herb-Crusted Salmon with Steamed Broccoli and Quinoa

Snack: Veggie Sticks with Hummus

Dessert: Greek Yogurt Berry Parfait

Breakfast: Veggie Omelette with Whole Grain Toast

Lunch: Grilled Chicken Salad with Quinoa

Dinner: Grilled Lemon Herb Chicken with Roasted Vegetables

Snack: Greek Yogurt with Berries and Almonds

Dessert: Baked Apples with Cinnamon and Walnuts

DAY 4

Breakfast: Greek Yogurt Parfait with Berries and Nuts

Lunch: Baked Salmon with Roasted Vegetables

Dinner: Baked Herb-Crusted Salmon with Steamed Broccoli and Quinoa

Snack: Veggie Sticks with Hummus

Dessert: Greek Yogurt Berry Parfait

Breakfast: Veggie Omelette with Whole Grain Toast

Lunch: Grilled Chicken Salad with Quinoa

Dinner: Grilled Lemon Herb Chicken with Roasted Vegetables

Snack: Greek Yogurt with Berries and Almonds

Dessert: Baked Apples with Cinnamon and Walnuts

Breakfast: Greek Yogurt Parfait with Berries and Nuts

Lunch: Baked Salmon with Roasted Vegetables

Dinner: Baked Herb-Crusted Salmon with Steamed Broccoli and Quinoa

Snack: Veggie Sticks with Hummus

Dessert: Greek Yogurt Berry Parfait

DAY 7

Breakfast: Veggie Omelette with Whole Grain Toast

Lunch: Grilled Chicken Salad with Quinoa

Dinner: Grilled Lemon Herb Chicken with Roasted Vegetables

Snack: Greek Yogurt with Berries and Almonds

Dessert: Baked Apples with Cinnamon and Walnuts

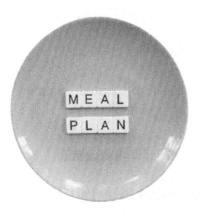

CONCLUSION

Understanding and managing glycemic load is a pivotal step toward fostering healthier dietary habits, especially for individuals seeking to regulate blood sugar levels and promote overall well-being. This comprehensive guide has unveiled a myriad of low to moderate glycemic foods across various categories, empowering readers with the knowledge to make informed choices for healthier eating.

By delving into the nuances of glycemic load and its impact on health, we've explored the intricate differences between glycemic load and glycemic index, providing a deeper understanding of how these factors influence our body's response to carbohydrates. We've navigated through the basics, examining factors affecting glycemic load in foods and highlighting its pivotal role in effective diet planning.

From breakfast to dinner, snack time to dessert, this guide has curated a diverse array of recipes, offering delicious and practical options that prioritize lower glycemic choices without compromising on taste or satisfaction.

These recipes, coupled with portion sizes and nutritional details, serve as valuable tools in crafting meals that harmonize with blood sugar management goals.

Furthermore, the exploration of high-glycemic foods and their effects on blood sugar levels has shed light on foods to limit or avoid, empowering individuals to make conscious decisions about their dietary intake.

Ultimately, this guide aims to inspire a balanced approach to nutrition, emphasizing the significance of incorporating low to moderate glycemic foods into everyday meals. By embracing these principles, readers can embark on a journey towards a healthier lifestyle, one mindful choice at a time. As the understanding of glycemic load continues to evolve, may this resource stand as a steadfast companion in fostering healthier eating habits and promoting better overall health for all.

WEEKLY MEAL PLANNER JOURNAL

WEEK ——————— MONTH ———————

MONDAY

SATURDAY

TUESDAY

SUNDAY

WEDNESDAY

SHOPPING LIST

- ◯ _____
- ◯ _____
- ◯ _____
- ◯ _____
- ◯ _____
- ◯ _____
- ◯ _____
- ◯ _____

THURSDAY

FRIDAY

NOTES:

- ◯ _____
- ◯ _____
- ◯ _____
- ◯ _____

WEEKLY MEAL PLANNER JOURNAL

WEEK _____   MONTH _____

MONDAY

SATURDAY

TUESDAY

SUNDAY

WEDNESDAY

SHOPPING LIST

○ _____
○ _____
○ _____
○ _____
○ _____
○ _____
○ _____
○ _____

THURSDAY

FRIDAY

NOTES:

○ _____
○ _____
○ _____
○ _____

WEEKLY MEAL PLANNER JOURNAL

WEEK _____ MONTH _____

MONDAY

SATURDAY

TUESDAY

SUNDAY

WEDNESDAY

SHOPPING LIST

- ○ _____
- ○ _____
- ○ _____
- ○ _____

THURSDAY

- ○ _____
- ○ _____
- ○ _____
- ○ _____

FRIDAY

NOTES:

- ○ _____
- ○ _____
- ○ _____
- ○ _____

WEEKLY MEAL PLANNER JOURNAL

WEEK _____ MONTH _____

MONDAY

SATURDAY

TUESDAY

SUNDAY

WEDNESDAY

SHOPPING LIST

- ○ _____
- ○ _____
- ○ _____
- ○ _____
- ○ _____
- ○ _____
- ○ _____
- ○ _____

THURSDAY

FRIDAY

NOTES:

- ○ _____
- ○ _____
- ○ _____
- ○ _____

WEEKLY MEAL PLANNER JOURNAL

WEEK _____   MONTH _____

MONDAY

TUESDAY

WEDNESDAY

THURSDAY

FRIDAY

SATURDAY

SUNDAY

SHOPPING LIST

- ○ _____
- ○ _____
- ○ _____
- ○ _____
- ○ _____
- ○ _____
- ○ _____
- ○ _____

NOTES:

- ○ _____
- ○ _____
- ○ _____
- ○ _____

WEEKLY MEAL PLANNER JOURNAL

WEEK _____   MONTH _____

| MONDAY | SATURDAY |

| TUESDAY | SUNDAY |

| WEDNESDAY | SHOPPING LIST |

| THURSDAY |

| FRIDAY | NOTES: |

WEEKLY MEAL PLANNER JOURNAL

WEEK _____ MONTH _____

MONDAY	SATURDAY

TUESDAY	SUNDAY

WEDNESDAY	SHOPPING LIST

- ○ _____
- ○ _____
- ○ _____
- ○ _____
- ○ _____
- ○ _____
- ○ _____
- ○ _____

THURSDAY

FRIDAY

NOTES:

- ○ _____
- ○ _____
- ○ _____
- ○ _____

WEEKLY MEAL PLANNER JOURNAL

WEEK ——————— MONTH ———————

MONDAY

SATURDAY

TUESDAY

SUNDAY

WEDNESDAY

SHOPPING LIST

- ○ ——————————
- ○ ——————————
- ○ ——————————
- ○ ——————————

THURSDAY

- ○ ——————————
- ○ ——————————
- ○ ——————————
- ○ ——————————

FRIDAY

NOTES:
- ○ ——————————
- ○ ——————————
- ○ ——————————
- ○ ——————————

WEEKLY MEAL PLANNER
JOURNAL

WEEK ——————— MONTH ———————

MONDAY

SATURDAY

TUESDAY

SUNDAY

WEDNESDAY

SHOPPING LIST

○ ——————————
○ ——————————
○ ——————————
○ ——————————
○ ——————————
○ ——————————
○ ——————————
○ ——————————

THURSDAY

FRIDAY

NOTES:

○ ——————————
○ ——————————
○ ——————————
○ ——————————

WEEKLY MEAL PLANNER JOURNAL

WEEK —————————— MONTH ——————————

MONDAY

SATURDAY

TUESDAY

SUNDAY

WEDNESDAY

SHOPPING LIST

- ○ ——————————
- ○ ——————————
- ○ ——————————
- ○ ——————————
- ○ ——————————
- ○ ——————————
- ○ ——————————
- ○ ——————————

THURSDAY

FRIDAY

NOTES:

- ○ ——————————
- ○ ——————————
- ○ ——————————
- ○ ——————————

Made in the USA
Monee, IL
15 October 2024

67842880R00148